SLIMMING WORLD's
CURRY FEAST

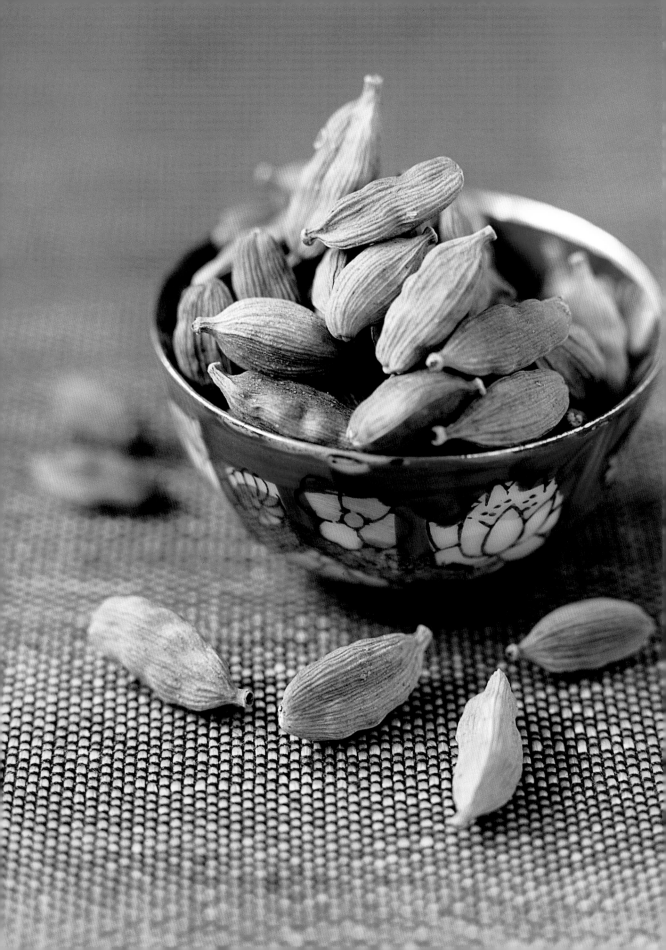

SLIMMING WORLD's
CURRY FEAST

120 mouth-watering Indian recipes to make at home

EBURY
PRESS

First published in 2006

10 9 8 7 6 5 4 3

First published by Ebury Press
Random House, 20 Vauxhall Bridge Road, London SW1V 2SA

Random House Australia (Pty) Limited
20 Alfred Street, Milsons Point, Sydney, New South Wales 2061, Australia

Random House New Zealand Limited
18 Poland Road, Glenfield, Auckland 10, New Zealand

Random House South Africa (Pty) Limited
Endulini, 5a Jubilee Road, Parktown 2193, South Africa

The Random House Group Limited
Reg. No. 954009

www.randomhouse.co.uk

A CIP catalogue record for this book is available from the British Library

ISBN 9 780091 90926 0

Recipes created by: Sunil Vijayakar
Editor: Emma Callery
Design: Nicky Barneby

Food photography: Jon Whitaker
Food stylist: Sunil Vijayakar
Props stylist: Rachel Jukes

For Slimming World
Founder and Chairman: Margaret Miles-Bramwell
Managing Director: Caryl Richards
Project co-ordinators: Allison Brentnall and Beverley Farnsworth
Text by Sara Niven

Printed and bound in China by C&C Offset Printing Co., Ltd.

SLIMMING WORLD

Founded in 1969 by Margaret Miles-Bramwell, Slimming World is the UK's most advanced slimming organisation. It currently manages 5,500 groups nationwide, with over 250,000 members attending every month, and another 15,000 attending free of charge as successful target members. Each week, around 2,000 members reach their personal target weight. Slimming World's unique approach to weight loss is an extraordinary success story.

COOKERY NOTES

* *Both metric and imperial measures are given for the recipes. Follow either set of measures as they are not interchangeable.*

* *All spoon measures are level: 1 tsp = 5ml spoon, 1 tbsp = 15ml spoon.*

* ⓥ *Suitable for vegetarians*

* ❋ *Suitable for freezing*

* *Ovens should be preheated to the specified temperature. Grills should also be preheated.*

* *Use large eggs unless otherwise specified.*

* *Note that some of the recipes contain lightly cooked eggs. Avoid serving these to anyone who is pregnant or in a vulnerable health group, because of the small risk of salmonella infection.*

* *Always use fresh herbs, unless dried herbs are suggested in the recipe.*

* *Use freshly ground black pepper and sea salt unless otherwise specified.*

CONTENTS

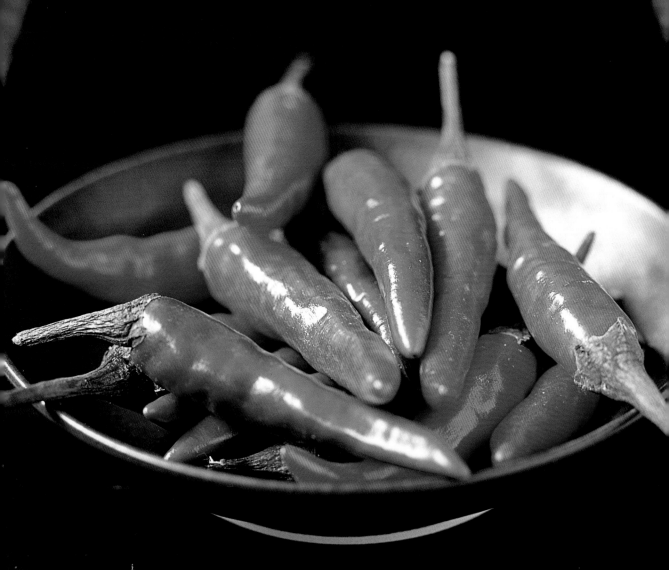

FOREWORD

Dear Reader,

A heartfelt and warm welcome to the latest addition to Slimming World's enticing collection of recipe books, Slimming World's Curry Feast. They say that variety is the spice of life. Well, in this book you'll find that spice adds the variety and the flavour to dozens of dishes, from favourite classic curries to delicate and unusual accompaniments – and they're all great for your slimming campaign!

If you have bought this book because you love spicy food and are always looking for new ideas, that's wonderful. And if you're looking for a way to enjoy your favourite meals without worrying about what they might do to your waistline, that's even better! Because what makes this cookery book special is that all the recipes have been designed to fit in with our famous Food Optimising, Slimming World's unique eating plan that makes it easy to lose weight without ever having to feel hungry or deprive yourself of foods you love. Like everything about Slimming World, it's about people who love life and want to live it to the max!

At Slimming World we have over 36 years' experience of understanding slimmers and helping them to manage their weight – driven by a passionate belief that people who are overweight have enough of a burden to carry; we do not need the added weight of guilt and low self-esteem compounded by so many rigid, uncompromising and boring diet regimes.

That's why Slimming World is based on freedom: freedom to choose what you eat instead of following a limited diet sheet; freedom to decide the size you want to be and how quickly you want to reach it; freedom to choose the type and amount of physical activity in your life; and most of all – freedom to be yourself, in a warm, supportive Slimming World group that will not judge you, nag you or make you feel like anything other than the wonderful, confident, valuable individual that you are.

It's powerful stuff, freedom – more exhilarating than the spiciest curry! And as hundreds of thousands of successful Slimming World members have found, that powerful feeling of liberation from guilt and despair around food, that soaring self-esteem, can take you to places beyond your dreams, let alone your expectations.

It's virtually impossible to express that kind of power on paper, so this book can only offer a brief insight into everything Slimming World has to offer, because what we have to offer is mega! It's sensational, exceptional and revolutionary and it's unique to Slimming World. So, like the recipes themselves, this book will give you a taste of something new and something 'more-ish'.

Slimming World's Curry Feast could simply provide you with some great-tasting recipes that prove healthy, non-fattening food can be exciting, or it could change your life – by opening the door to Slimming World. However you choose to use it, I'm delighted to welcome you into our world.

And if your weight is an issue for you, and you are thinking, 'If only I could find something I could stick to that would work for me,' let me promise you, from the bottom of my heart, that Slimming World and Food Optimising are what you've been looking for. Come and join us, and together we'll start that first step of your amazing journey to success.

With love,

Margaret Miles-Bramwell
Slimming World's Founder and Chairman

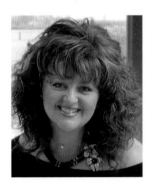

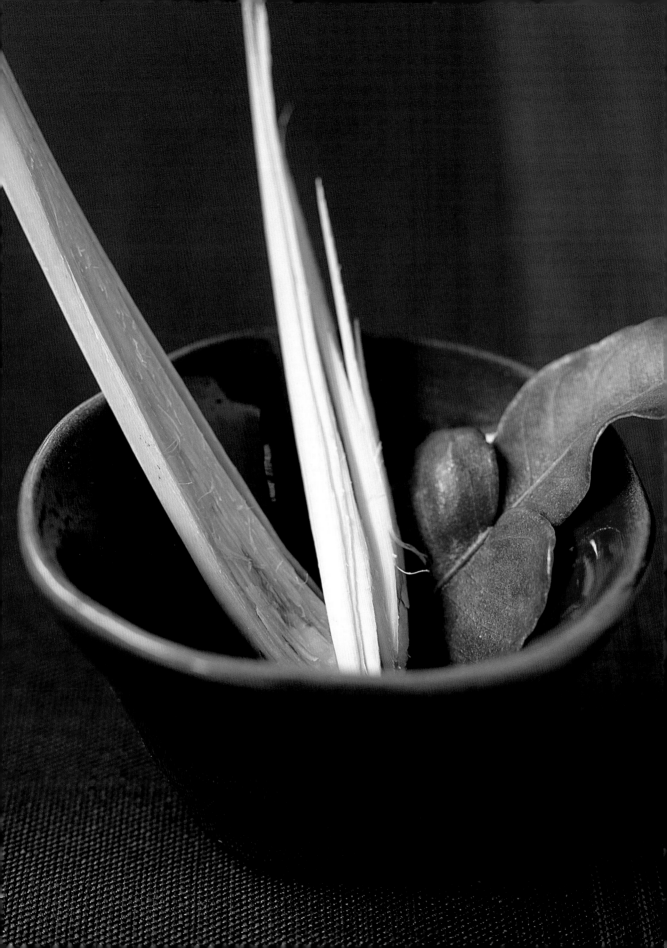

OPTIMISE YOUR LIFE

If you're reading this, there's a good chance you are a curry lover – or know someone who is! Before now, you might have seen this as a bit of a guilty secret or something that could never fit in with healthy eating.

This book will prove otherwise, we promise! It shows you how to prepare quick and easy meals including main dishes, potato and rice accompaniments, and explains how these recipes can be incorporated into Slimming World's unique Food Optimising plan to enable you to lose weight healthily and easily. You may already be familiar with Food Optimising or you may never have heard of it before. Either way this book is for you!

If you don't want to lose weight, then this book will show you how to cook great-tasting, healthy, authentic Asian dishes at a fraction of the cost of takeaways or restaurant meals. And if you would like to lose weight, then you'll also get a real insight into a healthy eating plan that is working right now for hundreds of thousands of Slimming World members in groups all over the country.

Food Optimising is a different way of thinking about food, removing the guilt from eating – and that applies to curries, cottage pie or carrot cake! The emphasis is firmly on using healthy foods to fill you up, based on the unique concept of 'Free Foods', which are foods that you can eat completely freely! Many of the recipes in this book are just that – Free! – meaning you can enjoy seconds, thirds, even fourths if you can find the room – without a moment's thought or guilt.

> **Slimming World's Food Optimising is based on the following basic principles:**
> * That we enjoy eating good food.
> * That we want to eat until we feel full.
> * That we want to continue to enjoy a social life while slimming.
> * That we want to be treated like adults and given choices.

A SLIMMING SUCCESS STORY

In the following chapters you'll find out more about the amazing concept of Food Optimising:

* You'll **learn** why losing weight the Slimming World way means an end to faddy diets and tiny portions.
* You'll **discover** that you really can eat your fill of all kinds of delicious meals, without worrying about weighing or measuring a thing.
* And you'll be **thrilled** to find that you can do all this and still lose weight healthily, as many thousands of slimmers have already discovered for themselves with Food Optimising. Each week around 250,000 members attend one of Slimming World's 5,500 groups nationwide, with 15,000 attending free of charge as successful target members and 2,000 slimmers reaching their personal target weight.

Given the choice, who wouldn't want to be slim and healthy? That needn't mean being a certain weight or clothes size – attractive, healthy bodies come in all shapes and sizes.

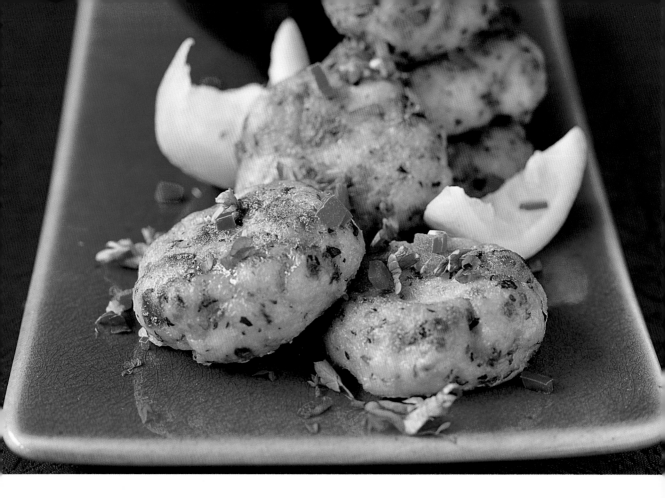

It's about having a body that moves lightly and easily, a shape that 'fits in' wherever we might find ourselves, and the energy to enjoy life to the full. And who wouldn't rather achieve this through healthy, enjoyable eating and a moderate amount of activity, than by starvation and faddy diets?

The problem slimmers have come up against in the past is that they have been asked to choose between their natural enjoyment of food and their desire to lose weight. With celebrities telling us about their one-meal-a-day diet and other slimming programmes advocating giving up entire food groups – even basics like milk and potatoes – it's not surprising that slimming has been seen as a sacrifice. And while we can all make a sacrifice when we have to, who wants to live their life that way?

That's precisely the reason why so many people delay taking action about their weight or lose it, only to put it back on – because the methods of slimming they've followed in the past are not something they find realistic to keep up in the long term, so they start feeling bored, hungry or both.

People beat themselves up for being weak-willed when yet another dieting attempt goes wrong, yet few stop to consider that they didn't fail the diet; the diet failed them!

* Perhaps they eat out a lot and the restrictive regime doesn't account for this?
* Perhaps they have a sweet tooth but chocolate, cakes and desserts are banned?
* Or maybe they enjoy a glass of wine with dinner, which is not allowed for.
* Perhaps they have limited time to prepare special meals, or have a passion for so-called

'fattening' dishes such as curries – which, having picked up this book, the chances are you'll share!

The founder of Slimming World, Margaret Miles-Bramwell, has herself struggled with all of these issues. She began to realise that most weight loss plans were fatally flawed, for the simple reason that they weren't food-friendly or people-friendly!

The trend in the Seventies and Eighties for diets that restricted slimmers to just a few food groups or even just a couple of foods (remember all those grapefruit, pineapples and eggs?) is a good example. They were boring and terrible for your social life, but it was worse than that; diets like these that severely limit your calorie intake are counter-productive for long-term weight management. This is partly because they do nothing to encourage the permanent, sustainable changes in lifestyle that are needed to get slim and stay slim; as soon as normal eating habits are resumed, the weight goes back on.

It is also now known that severely restricting food intake by crash dieting can result in the loss of lean tissue (such as muscle) from the body as well as body fat. Loss of lean tissue slows the metabolic rate (the rate at which the body uses up energy) making it harder to lose weight and stay slim in the long term. This is why gradual weight loss on a sensible calorie intake is the ideal for getting and staying slim healthily – exactly what Food Optimising does.

Ever since Slimming World was launched in 1969, Food Optimising has ensured that

Free to eat, free to be you

Food Optimising is very different from any kind of weight loss plan you may have encountered before.

* For one thing, it actively encourages you to eat, whenever and wherever you like! Fancy a cooked breakfast with all the trimmings? That's fine – and it's also fine if you're not a 'full English' fan. You can go out for meals and enjoy socialising – and you don't have to pretend biscuits and chocolate no longer exist!

* Within the basic guidelines of Food Optimising, you are free to satisfy your appetite with hundreds of different foods in unlimited amounts. And you can tantalise your taste buds with any food you like – no food is on the 'banned' list at Slimming World.

* It's no wonder that many Slimming World members find that they are actually eating far more since they started Food Optimising than they were before. The difference is that they are actually losing weight.

members benefit from the latest research into weight management, healthy eating and lifestyle change. The basic principles and the reasoning behind it have remained the same because it is a way of eating that is endorsed by nutritionists and because hundreds of thousands of successful slimmers have proved that it works. Not just as a 'quick fix', but as a way of continuing to enjoy eating healthily and normally and staying slim for life.

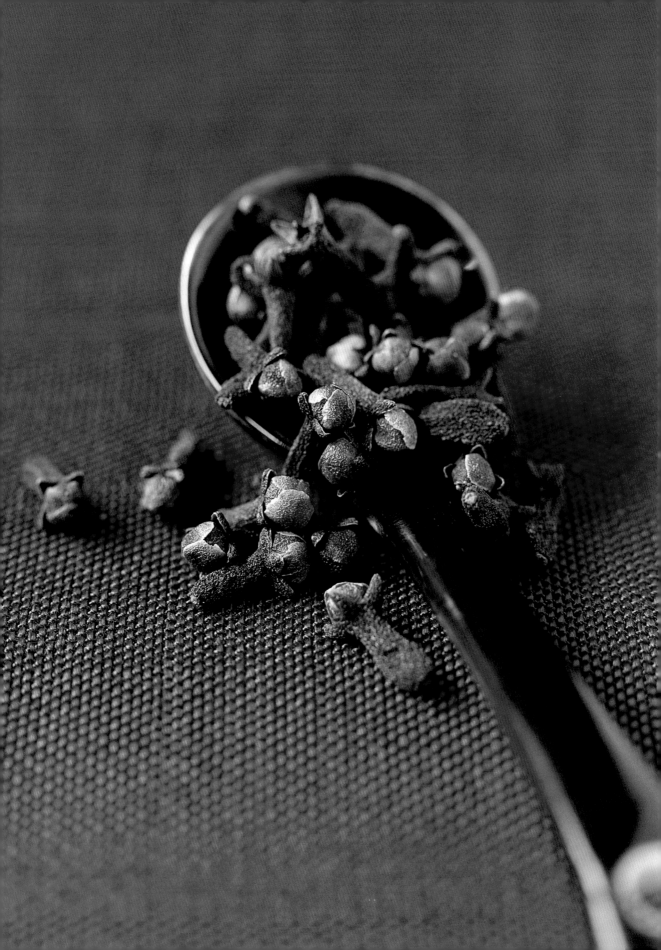

USE YOUR CHOICE POWER

Food Optimising is all about choice. Slimming World members are adults who don't need to be told what to eat and when to eat it. The best person for knowing what you fancy to eat and when you fancy it is you!

There's no being bossed around, because you are the boss. Which is why we call our Slimming World clubs 'groups' and the people who run them 'Consultants', not teachers or leaders. Yes, you'll learn plenty at Slimming World but you'll be an active part of that learning process and your Consultant will be there to advise, support and encourage, not to tell you what they think you should do or to browbeat you into doing it.

THE CHOICE IS YOURS

* You decide what you eat, when you eat it and, nearly always, how much you eat.
* You decide how you want to deal with social occasions where tempting food will be on offer.
* You decide how much weight you'd like to lose and how long you'd like to take doing it.
* In short:
  YOU are in control!

One of the main things you will be in control of is deciding which Food Optimising choice to follow. You can do this on a daily basis or even meal by meal, so you can change around as often as you'd like. Or if you find a routine that suits you, you can simply stick with that. Again, the choice is yours. Food Optimising is devised to fit around you, not the other way round.

Slimming World offers members four choices, which are all part of the Food Optimising plan. These are:

* Green
* Original
* Mix2Max
* Success Express

Before looking at each option, it's helpful to look at one factor all four choices have in common. This is one of the foundation stones that Slimming World is built on. It is also one of the reasons so many Slimming World members succeed in losing weight and keeping it off. That's the principle of Free Foods.

FREE FOR ALL

Free Foods are foods that you can eat freely (hence the name!) in unlimited amounts, whenever and wherever you want. They are wholesome, everyday foods that you don't need to weigh, measure or feel guilty about eating. In fact you can feel positively virtuous when it comes to eating your fill of Free Food fruit and vegetables as they are great providers of vitamins, minerals and fibre.

Which foods are Free depends partly on what choice you are following. For example carbohydrate-rich foods like potatoes, pasta and rice are Free Foods on the Green choice while on the Original choice Free Foods are rich in protein and include lean meat, poultry and fish. We'll explain this in more detail later. There are also some foods that are Free whatever choice you are following, which for this reason are called Superfree Foods.

With these foods (see box, below), you can eat your fill from whichever of the four choices you are following.

With all these foods you are actively encouraged to eat as much as you want to satisfy your appetite. Healthy eating guidelines recommend we eat at least five servings of fruit and vegetables a day to stay healthy but as so many of them are Free Foods when Food Optimising you can enjoy even more – as many servings as you like in fact!

Eating lots of fruit and vegetables will fill you up, and will actively benefit your health as well – many Slimming World members say they didn't realise how few fruit and vegetables they used to eat before starting Food Optimising.

Even Food Optimisers who previously avoided 'eating their greens' have found that once they are aware of all the different Free fruits and vegetables and all the delicious and imaginative Slimming World recipes, they end up trying and liking far more than they expected to!

FREE THINKING

If you are used to calorie-counting diets it can be difficult to get used to the idea of Free Foods. How is it possible to lose weight eating unlimited amounts of foods like chicken or potatoes, without counting calories?

The answer is you can; there really is no catch. Chicken is a Free Food on the **Original** choice, which is based on eating your fill of protein-rich foods such as meat, fish and poultry. Potatoes cooked without fat are Free Foods on the **Green** choice, along with rice, pasta and pulses. The reason foods are Free or Superfree (Free on both Green and Original) is because Food Optimising works on the principle of the ability of foods to satisfy appetite, rather than the amount you eat.

Food Optimising is based on scientific studies, including research pioneered and funded by Slimming World, into whether certain kinds of food are better at satisfying and filling us up than others. The results have clearly shown that foods rich in protein or carbohydrate are the most satiating (best at satisfying the appetite) while fat is the least satiating of the food groups. Research at Leeds University, in which test groups of volunteers were encouraged to eat freely, found that when

THE FABULOUS FOUR

Having looked at the principles of Free Food, it's time to look in a bit more detail at the four fabulous choices that make up Food Optimising. As well as the popular Green and Original choices, at the start of 2005 two new Food Optimising choices were introduced – Mix2Max and Success Express – to give Slimming World members even greater freedom of choice and rate of weight loss.

The Green choice

On the Green choice you will eat lots of filling, healthy carbohydrate-rich foods, plus generous, measured servings of protein-rich foods. Comforting foods like potatoes, rice, dried pasta, baked beans, peas and lentils are all Free Foods on Green, while you can enjoy lean meat, poultry, fish and seafood as Healthy Extras (see page 18). And of course you can eat unlimited Superfree Foods from the list opposite. If you love giant jacket potatoes, vegetable curry or chilli with a pile of rice, or a massive Spanish omelette with potatoes and onions, then the Green choice is for you! Another typical Green choice meal would be a huge plate of pasta with a rich, chunky ratatouille sauce, sprinkled with Parmesan cheese and served with broccoli and a wholemeal roll, followed by a large fresh fruit salad with very low fat fruit yogurt. Add a glass of red wine (see The Sense Behind Syns, page 19) and you'll find it impossible to believe you're slimming!

The Original choice

On the Original choice the balance of your plate is reversed so that you enjoy unlimited amounts of lean meat, poultry, fish and seafood with measured portions of carbohydrate-rich foods such as pasta, potatoes, beans and pulses. The Original choice is great for meat lovers who want plenty of bacon for breakfast and fancy going to town on turkey or tucking into a massive juicy steak for lunch. Imagine being at a barbecue and being able to eat your fill of chicken, beef and fish knowing you'll still lose weight that week! You can also have your fill of Superfree Foods so if you'd like a big plate of roasted peppers and onions with your kebab, eggs with your morning bacon or want to round off your steak supper with strawberries and very low fat natural yogurt, go right ahead! And of course you can continue to have a decent-sized portion of carbohydrate-rich food in the form of potatoes, pasta or pulses to accompany your fish or meat feast.

Mix2Max

Mix2Max is a way of mixing Green and Original choices for maximum flexibility. Instead of sticking to Green or Original meals all day you can make your choice at each mealtime, and snack on Superfree Foods in between. Max2Max is fantastic if you're not sure what you'll be eating at each meal and want to keep your options open.

Success Express

Success Express is a way of boosting your weight loss that doesn't involve any weighing or measuring and is based on a straightforward Two to One principle: at each meal, fill two-thirds of your plate with Superfree Foods, and on the remaining third of your plate have your choice of foods that are Free on Green OR Original. It's easy to follow, gets you focused on Free and Superfree Foods, and is a super-healthy, no-nonsense way of planning your meals.

their diet was secretly controlled to provide a high carbohydrate/low fat diet the volunteers lost weight, despite eating whatever they wanted. This was in contrast to the week when they were given high fat/low carbohydrate foods, when they all put on weight.

Some members join Slimming World determined to test this principle to the limit! They eat as much Free Food as they possibly can, determined to be the exception that proves the rule. It's a great way of demonstrating to themselves that Free really means just that – when they see the weight coming off every week, they find it a thoroughly liberating experience!

The concept of Free Food is liberating from an emotional point of view as well. Knowing that food isn't 'rationed' when you're Food Optimising, and that there is no danger of running out of your daily allowance by teatime (or sooner!) helps to remove the tension and obsession over the next meal that so often accompanies rigid dieting regimes. With no strict rules to rebel against, Slimming World members behave like the discerning adults they are, instead of the naughty children many 'experts' think slimmers are. Knowing that you can eat a whole roast chicken doesn't mean that you will! But it does mean that it becomes much easier to relax around food and to develop a natural relationship with it – in fact, to eat just like slim people do.

WHICH TO CHOOSE?

As a new member of Slimming World, you will find that you lose weight easily and enjoyably

following 'Green days' or 'Original days' (see box, page 17): as the name suggests, you decide whether to go Green or Original and follow that choice all day. You can choose Green every day or have a mixture of Green and Original; it's up to you. Once you have been Food Optimising for a while, you might like to try Mix2Max or Success Express; your Consultant will be able to explain more about these options and how to make them work for you.

HEALTHY EXTRAS = EXTRA HEALTHY FOR YOU!

As well as all the Free Foods that are available on each choice, Food Optimisers choose every day from lists of Healthy Extras that include hundreds of foods such as milk, cheese, bread and cereals.

Healthy Extras ensure you get everything you need for a healthy balanced diet by providing a daily intake of foods rich in fibre, vitamins and minerals. Each day, Slimming World members make one or two selections from the list of

Healthy Extra 'a' choices include milk and cheese and have been selected because they are high in calcium, a mineral that's essential for good health and, recent research indicates, may also play a part in boosting weight loss.

Some Healthy Extra 'b' choices are high in fibre, which is vital for good digestion, and others contain important nutrients for a balanced diet. Examples include certain cereals, bread and some soups.

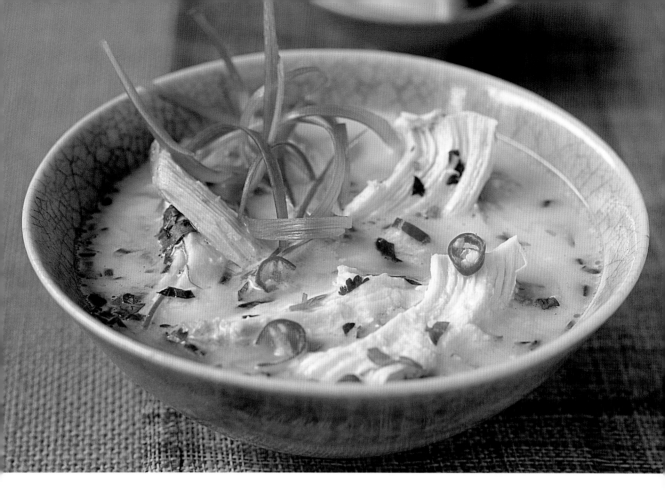

Healthy Extra 'a' choices and two selections from the Healthy Extra 'b' choices.

With so many Healthy Extras to choose from, Food Optimisers love to ring the changes to ensure maximum variety so that they never get bored – one of the keys to a healthy diet. Details of new food products that qualify as a Healthy Extra – such as the launch of a low-fat cheese or high-fibre cereal – are regularly available for Slimming World members so there is always something different to try.

THE SENSE BEHIND SYNS

The word Syn may sound like something we do when we can't bear a restrictive diet regime any more but the simple fact is that at Slimming World there are no saints or sinners – only human beings! 'Syn' actually comes from 'synergy', which according to the dictionary is what happens when 'the combined effects of certain elements exceed the sum of their individual effects.'

Together with Free Foods and Healthy Extras, Syns are the third element that makes Food Optimising so easy to stick to and such a healthy way of losing weight. Having an allowance of Syns each day provides the perfect combination of 'freewheeling and control' – creating a non-restrictive healthy eating plan that allows for the fact that most of us enjoy a glass of wine, slice of cake or packet of crisps. Some diet plans require you to count every calorie you eat, but without differentiating between lettuce and lard in terms of what's good for you. Food Optimising ensures your focus is on filling, nutritious Free Foods and Healthy Extras, with Syns on hand to account

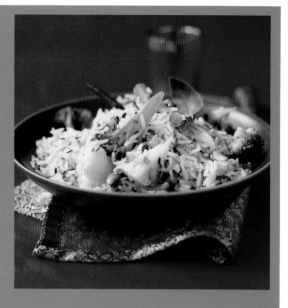

AT A GLANCE

* **Food Optimising** is the name given to Slimming World's healthy eating plan.
* There are four choices in the plan – you can choose a different one to follow each day or stick to the same one depending on your eating habits and preference.
* **The Green Choice** is based on enjoying pasta, potatoes, rice and pulses in unlimited quantities with measured portions of meat and fish.
* **The Original Choice** is based on enjoying meat, poultry and fish in unlimited quantities with measured portions of pasta, potatoes and pulses.
* **Mix2Max** and **SuccessExpress** are two new choices based on the same basic Food Optimising principles but with even more freedom of choice; your Consultant can explain more about how these work.
* **Free Foods** are enjoyed in unlimited amounts on the Green or Original choice.
* **Superfree Foods** are foods that can be enjoyed in unlimited amounts while following any of the plans.
* **Healthy Extras** are foods that are high in fibre, vitamins or minerals.
* **Syns** are the extras that ensure you can still enjoy your favourite foods.

for those 'bits on the side' such as ketchup, gravy or mayonnaise, or the little extras that we enjoy as snacks, desserts or when eating out.

If a food isn't Free or a Healthy Extra on a particular choice, then it has a Syn value. The number of Syns Food Optimisers have each day can vary, but on average most people find 10 Syns a day works well.

OPTIMISE YOUR HEALTH

If you ever feel confused trying to keep up with the latest healthy eating advice, that's one less thing to worry about when you start Food Optimising! Slimming World's nutrition experts keep us constantly updated with the latest in thoroughly researched healthy eating information and ensure it is incorporated into all of Food Optimising's choices, so members lose weight effectively while not just safeguarding their health, but actively boosting it.

One example of this is the way in which Food Optimising actively encourages members to make the most of readily available fresh foods. While cooking every meal from scratch is not an essential part of Food Optimising, members often find that they are tempted into the kitchen to make delicious Free Food meals, using our wide selection of quick, easy Slimming World recipes. Cooking at home saves money as well as Syns, and it is also a great opportunity for cutting back on fat, sugar and salt as you become more aware of what goes in the food that you are eating.

By Food Optimising fully and including plenty of Free Foods every day, you will automatically be eating a balanced diet containing all the nutrients needed for optimum health. In other words, a diet that's high in fibre, low in fat, with the right balance of protein and carbohydrates and enough vitamins and minerals to provide your body with everything it needs to function at its best.

Doing something about being overweight is obviously beneficial to health but doing it in a way that deprives your body of essential nutrients is anything but. It is not enough simply to promise a weight loss – Slimming World members know that in addition they will be eating in a way that benefits their health in both the short and long term:

SHORT-TERM BENEFITS

Not long after starting Food Optimising you may notice some of the following:

* An increase in energy levels.
* Improved digestion.
* Improved skin and a general healthy glow.
* Better quality of sleep.

LONG-TERM BENEFITS

Over time, losing weight with Food Optimising can help you stay healthy in many important ways:

* Maintaining bone strength to reduce the risk of osteoporosis.
* Reducing risk of developing Type 2 diabetes.
* Reducing risk of developing certain cancers.
* Reducing risk of heart disease and strokes.
* Relief from joint problems such as osteoarthritis.
* Reduction of high blood pressure.

What's more, you do not need to have reached your ideal weight for these health benefits to start to take effect. If you are very overweight, losing just 10% of your starting weight and keeping it off can make a significant and beneficial difference to a whole range of conditions. Slimming World recognises this with **Club 10**, a reward scheme that celebrates the success of every member who reaches this milestone and maintains their loss – or goes on to lose even more – over at least 10 weeks.

Many members with medical conditions report that losing weight with Slimming World has significantly reduced the symptoms they suffer, meaning that they need less medication than before and have improved mobility. Some even find they no longer need the operation they had previously been told was necessary.

Our firm belief is that the best thing to do is to slim while eating in a way that is proven to have numerous beneficial effects and this is just what Food Optimising does. After all, we want to live long, healthy lives to make the most of our fabulous new slim bodies and extra energy!

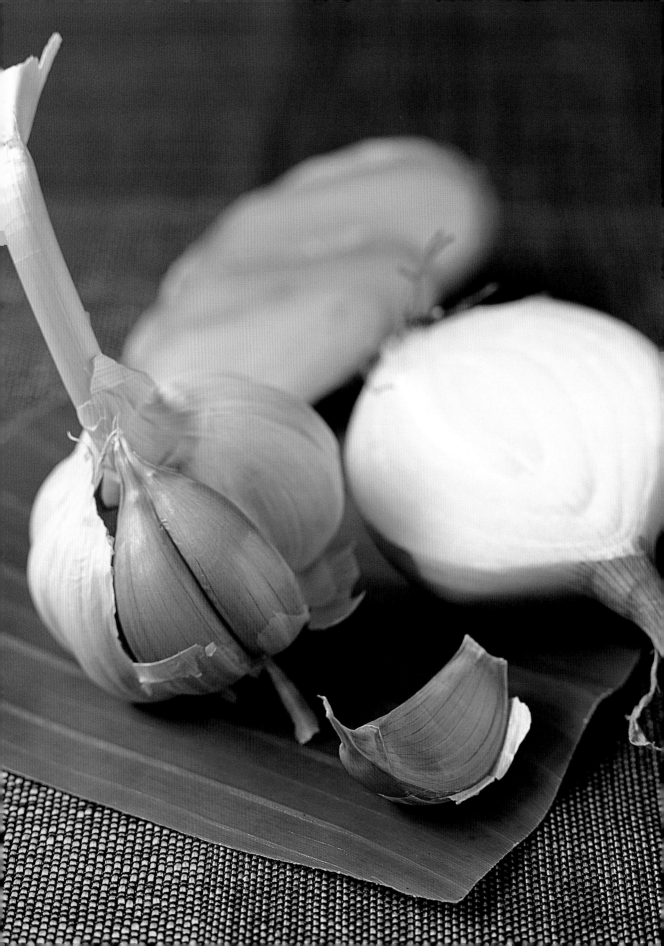

SLIMMING WORLD SYNERGY

The reason why Food Optimising is so effective is about more than the fact that you never need to go hungry or deny yourself your favourite foods. It also owes a great deal of its power to **synergy**. As mentioned on pages 19–20, this is the process of combining the right individual elements together to produce one powerful result.

Slimming World's synergy is based on three elements.

These are:

* **Food Optimising**: the eating plan that uses the synergy of Free Foods, Healthy Extras and Syns for fantastic results.
* **Image Therapy**: the powerful, exhilarating environment within a Slimming World group, that provides the support, encouragement and motivation members need to achieve their goals.
* **Body Magic**: a unique programme designed to encourage members to reap the numerous benefits of becoming more active – which doesn't have to mean going anywhere near a gym!

WORKING TOGETHER

Losing weight isn't just about what we eat; it is about the balance of energy in our lives and the way we see and think about ourselves. Body Magic takes care of the exercise side of the balance of energy and Image Therapy deals with our self-esteem and perceptions.

Image Therapy (Image stands for Individual Motivation and Group Experience) is unique to Slimming World and has been shown to have a powerful effect in helping members fulfil their potential.

To get an idea of how it works, it might help to imagine a time when you have looked at your reflection in the mirror on a bad day (this is probably quite easy as it happens to us all!).

Perhaps you notice small lines around your eyes, decide your teeth aren't looking as white as you'd like and realise the top you're wearing isn't as flattering as you'd thought.

You might have walked away with a fairly negative view of your appearance as a result. Imagine then, spending time chatting to a small group of close friends and admitting how you are feeling. One comments on the fact that she loves the colour of your eyes and envies the fact that you don't have to wear glasses. Another tells you that the colour of the shirt you're wearing really suits you – while a third confides that she felt her teeth weren't as white as she'd like them either and suggests a toothpaste she found that really helped her. The next time you look in the mirror you see all the good points your friends have commented on – and you appreciate the advice about the toothpaste, as well as knowing that you're not the only one who worries about the colour of their teeth!

If you're wondering what on earth toothpaste has to do with slimming, imagine that you are at a Slimming World group meeting. Perhaps you've had a difficult week personally and are not feeling too good about yourself. Or you've discovered something that gets in your way each week – such as finding it hard saying no to the cake trolley at work – and wonder if others have had similar problems?

GROUPS ARE GREAT

A growing body of research suggests that when it comes to losing weight, people who take part in a group are more successful than those who go it alone. For this reason, group participation is regularly recommended by health professionals as part of a weight management programme. For example, The National Clinical Guidelines recommended for use in Scotland (SIGN) suggest a support scheme within a weight loss programme, and the British Dietetic Association has also pointed out that discussion groups and workshops are good ways in which people can learn, enjoy support, and draw on others' experiences.

Attending group sessions has also been established as being valuable in helping people maintain weight once they have lost it: a study into different methods of weight loss funded by the Department of Health and published in 1999 reported that attending a group was 'one of the most effective treatment components' in keeping weight off.

comfort-eat after receiving some upsetting news and want to know how others cope in similar circumstances. Or you may find yourself on the receiving end of praise from the group for a triumph you might not have even identified as one – such as staying the same weight in the week you had your birthday.

By acknowledging that we all have difficult days, suggesting ways of dealing with certain situations and focusing on positives, Image Therapy addresses the underlying issues that can lead to a weight problem in the first place – issues so many slimming programmes fail to address.

At Slimming World we know that it is simply not enough to tell people what to do and then wave them off, expecting fantastic results. Human beings need more than mere instructions – we need PRAISE: a sense of Pride, Reassurance, Affirmation, Inspiration, Support and Empathy.

Image Therapy provides all these things besides a sense of fun and friendship, and as a result of this group activity, each individual member benefits.

In Image Therapy, members are encouraged to share, confide and understand each other's weaknesses as well as celebrate each other's strengths. No-one is forced into disclosing anything they don't want to, but most members find it very hard to stay silent once they realise they are among friends – there is always so much to discuss!

You may have struggled with an urge to

MAGICAL MOVES

Along with Image Therapy, members will be introduced to another important ingredient in the special Slimming World 'synergy mix'. It's one that is tried and tested for results when it comes to losing weight and keeping it off. What's more, it is proven to bring about a whole host of other health benefits, besides giving you the kind of inner and outer

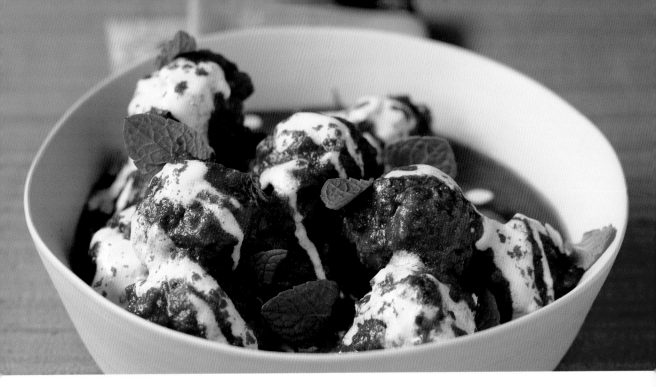

glow and feel-good factor that money can't buy.

Sounds pretty magical, doesn't it? That's why Slimming World calls it Body Magic. Body Magic is all about introducing more activity into our daily lives and reaping a whole host of benefits as a result. It's not about running marathons or climbing mountains – although amazingly as a result of Body Magic some of our members have done just these things and more!

We understand though that the longest journey starts with the smallest step and that's why Body Magic is about moving towards getting more active in a way that suits you and your lifestyle.

The benefits of exercise are so numerous we couldn't list them all here. But they can be divided into the following categories:

LOOKING GOOD

Regular activity has been proven to be a key factor in successfully maintaining weight loss. It burns energy, maintains muscles and raises metabolic rate. It improves circulation, giving your skin a boost and leaving you with the kind of natural glow make-up can't replicate. Depending on the type of exercise you do, you will also see the benefits as your body becomes toned and more shapely.

FEELING GREAT

When we exercise we produce endorphins, feel-good chemicals that give us a sense of wellbeing. This feel-good effect is so great that doctors can prescribe exercise in place of anti-depressants – regular, brisk 30-minute walks in the fresh air are thought to be particularly beneficial. There is evidence that exercise relieves symptoms of depression and anxiety (as well as reducing the risk of developing them), improves mood and raises self-esteem.

LIVING LONGER

There is plenty of strong evidence that regular physical activity contributes to a longer, healthier life by reducing the risk of various common disorders and protecting against conditions such as diabetes, osteoporosis and certain types of cancer, such as colon cancer. It also improves heart health and protects against heart disease, reduces the risk of stroke, helps build and maintain healthy bones and keeps joints mobile. It really is true that if you don't use it, you lose it!

Most of us know that regular exercise is a good thing. Yet despite all these fantastic benefits, only around 37 per cent of men and 25 per cent of women actually manage the recommended level of at least 30 minutes of moderately intensive exercise on at least five days a week.

Very often, it's psychological rather than physical barriers that hold us back from exercising – yet they can be just as challenging to overcome. Perhaps we feel guilty about the times we've joined a gym or a class and failed to keep going – another reminder of how 'useless' we are. Maybe we have memories of being humiliated on school sports days and have steered clear of anything 'athletic' ever since. Or it could just be so long since we did anything vaguely active that we worry about being embarrassed or physically unable to cope.

Sometimes we're just too tired! We may feel so shattered after a day at work or running around after the kids or both, that the thought of doing anything other than collapsing onto the couch at the end of the day leaves us cold.

Lack of time is another major reason for not exercising. We look at the '30 minutes five times a week' recommended guidelines given and wonder how we will manage to fit that into an already hectic schedule.

Yet all these factors (not excuses, because they are real concerns for people) can be addressed and that is exactly what Body Magic sets out to do. And just as Slimming World believes in giving members choice about what they eat and when, this approach also applies to exercise.

So if you hated PE at school, don't fancy the idea of spending precious time and money in a gym and wouldn't be seen dead jogging (or feel that you would probably end up that way if you did!), then Body Magic is not going to try to persuade you otherwise.

What it will do is show you alternatives to structured forms of exercise, ways of building up your fitness levels gradually and painlessly over time to make increased activity a way of life, and reward you for what you have achieved while providing a way of measuring just how far you've come.

Once you've started doing something and made that increased activity a habit, it becomes easy to motivate yourself to add a bit more – perhaps increasing a daily walk by another ten minutes, enjoying a weekly swim and sauna or trying out a dance class. Evidence has shown that building up activity levels gradually over time to make increased activity a habit means that you are far more likely to keep it up than if you throw yourself straight into a strenuous new exercise routine that quickly becomes too much.

It is never too late to start being physically active — even people who have been sedentary for years will benefit. If you already have a

BODY MAGIC IS THE SOLUTION

I don't have time

It might be true that finding an hour at a time for an exercise class, plus the time it would take to drive to a sports centre and back, might not be possible if you have a particularly busy life. But don't we all deserve at least an hour to ourselves each week? With a bit of planning, like finding someone to babysit or leaving work a bit earlier once or twice a week, could you manage it?

But walking the half mile and back to the paper shop instead of driving, taking the stairs at work instead of the lift and washing the car vigorously once a week are all effective ways of building increased activity into your lifestyle. Neither do you have to do the recommended 30 minutes of daily exercise in one go. When it comes to exercise, something is always better than nothing, so even if you just introduce a 15-minute daily walk into your routine, that's well worth doing. Do it twice a day, or spend 15 minutes dancing to a favourite record plus a further 15 doing energetic housework in the evening!

I'm too tired to exercise

It can be very difficult to find the motivation to do something active when you are genuinely shattered. Of course, if that's because you've been running around all day being active, that proves you've done a fair bit towards increased activity! But all too often after a long day we feel more exhausted and drained mentally than physically. And this is exactly the kind of tiredness that physical activity can help with. It might seem a huge effort to get off the couch, open the front door and walk round the block, but we can guarantee you will feel better for it. In fact, exercise is prescribed as a remedy for depression – the endorphins it produces give us a mental boost. And, of course, the fitter we get, the more energy we have.

It's years since I did anything – I wouldn't know how to start

With Body Magic, that's how. To start with, you'll work towards managing 45 minutes of activity each week, spread over at least three days and maintained for a month. Regularity rather than intensity is what counts, especially at the very beginning, so a few minutes of walking at a pace you can manage each day is an excellent start and far better than trying to do a full hour's exercise class in one go – then spending a fortnight getting over it!

Any activity, however small, is a start and will give you a foundation to build on. What's more, as someone who hasn't been active regularly you will notice the benefits of introducing more activity into your life more quickly than someone who is already fairly fit and working towards stepping up a level.

I have health problems and worry about starting any form of exercise

It is always good to consult your GP before starting an exercise programme and if you have a serious health concern, it is essential. But all GPs recognise the health benefits of increasing our activity levels and most will think it is a great idea that you are planning to do this gradually. You may not be encouraged to take up a high intensity activity such as squash if you have high blood pressure, but a brisk walk, swim or cycle ride will often get the seal of approval. Often, the right kind of moderate exercise can actively help alleviate certain conditions, such as lowering blood pressure and helping mobilise stiff joints.

chronic condition, being physically active can help reduce your symptoms – just check with your GP before starting an exercise programme. You do not need to do all of your activity at once, and the exercise does not need to be very vigorous for it to be beneficial.

THE BODY MAGIC AWARD SYSTEM

Body Magic is an activity programme, but it's about so much more than just burning up a few extra calories. With Body Magic, you'll be inspired to progress along the 'activity pathway' at your own pace, steadily building up the amount of activity in your life, enjoying the fun and sense of achievement that being active brings, and loving the benefits of having more energy, a more toned body and a year-round spring in your step! From a standing (or sitting) start to becoming fit for life, Body Magic will help you every step of the way.

There are four levels and awards – Bronze, Silver, Gold and Platinum. Everyone starts at the level they feel comfortable at, and gradually builds up their chosen activity or range of activities – remember, that can mean anything from martial arts to mowing the lawn – with the aim of moving on to the next level.

* You reach Bronze standard when you're enjoying 45 minutes of exercise a week, spread over at least three days and maintained for four weeks.
* Silver is yours when you've built up to six sessions of exercise of 15 minutes per week, spread over three to five days and maintained for four weeks.

* Now you're going for Gold! This means that you're now being active for ten 15-minute sessions a week spread over three to five days and maintained for eight weeks. This is the level that the Government recommends for maintaining general health.
* By now, you've got the fitness bug and you'll hardly notice you've reached Platinum standard – except that you feel so wonderful! You're at Platinum when activity has become part of your lifestyle and you're doing it for its own sake, not just to receive the rewards and praise at your Slimming World group (although they're great too!). Your Consultant can advise you when to aim for this level.

QUESTIONS AND ANSWERS

While reading through these chapters, you're likely to have questions: most people do when they are being introduced to a new concept for the first time! The best person to explain anything you're not clear about will be your Slimming World Consultant when you attend your first group meeting. In the meantime, here are the answers to two FAQs:

Q. I've tried lots of other diets and failed – usually because I gave in to temptation and ate my favourite foods. What's really so different about this one?
One crucial difference is that Food Optimising is not a 'diet'! It's a long-term healthy eating plan that can be followed for a lifetime, unlike restrictive regimes that most people can only follow for a few weeks at a time. Losing weight while eating plenty of filling, enjoyable meals

that you can actually look forward to, rather than just tolerate for a short time, is a world away from most people's experience of slimming.

The fact that you can eat out and enjoy foods often banned on diets, foods like chocolate, crisps and alcohol, is another of the main reasons slimmers succeed in losing and keeping weight off with Food Optimising.

At Slimming World we believe in the old adage, 'a little of what you fancy does you good' and Food Optimising is designed to make it easy for members to enjoy whatever that might be while still losing weight. Having a daily Syns allowance is the valuable safety net that ensures you never have to give up your favourite foods when you're Food Optimising. But we're all human, and sometimes a safety net isn't enough – we want to blow off steam and need a safety valve!

That's when Flexible Syns can help. They are Slimming World's way of ensuring that you never get that awful feeling that you've 'blown it' and that it's not worth carrying on. Flexible Syns are a way of staying in control in situations where you might otherwise lose it – without having to feel guilty or even make up for it afterwards. Your Consultant will explain how to use this most valuable tool that is the key to many, many members' long-term success.

And what if you do have a bad week, a bad month or even a bad year? No problem; it happens. No-one at Slimming World will judge you, so you need have no fears about returning to your group; and when you do go back, your Consultant and fellow members will be so pleased to see you that you'll feel you've never been away, and the emphasis will be on picking up where you have left off.

This emphasis on the positive rather than the negative is part of Slimming World's whole philosophy and many members have found that it makes all the difference to their success.

Q. How much weight can I expect to lose each week and how will I know what to aim for?
Everyone is different and people lose weight at different rates depending on factors including genetics, how active they are and how much weight they have to lose. When people start Food Optimising they often have some remarkable losses in the first week or two – as much as 3kg/7lbs or more – which of course is wonderfully motivating, and perfectly safe. By the time they have reached their target weight, their weight loss has usually averaged out at about 500g-1kg/1-2lbs each week, or 2-3.5kg/5-8lbs a month. This is a steady, healthy and sustainable rate of loss, so whether you start off with a big weight loss or take the slower route, you will get to where you want to be in the end.

At Slimming World your target weight is called your Personal Achievement Target (PAT) and it is exactly that – personal. No-one will tell you what weight to aim for, although your Consultant can advise you if you like; you don't have to set your PAT the moment you join Slimming World, and you can adjust it as you go. Once you have reached your PAT you can attend any Slimming World group anywhere, free of charge, for as long as you remain within 3lbs either side of your PAT – so that you are part of the Slimming World family for life!

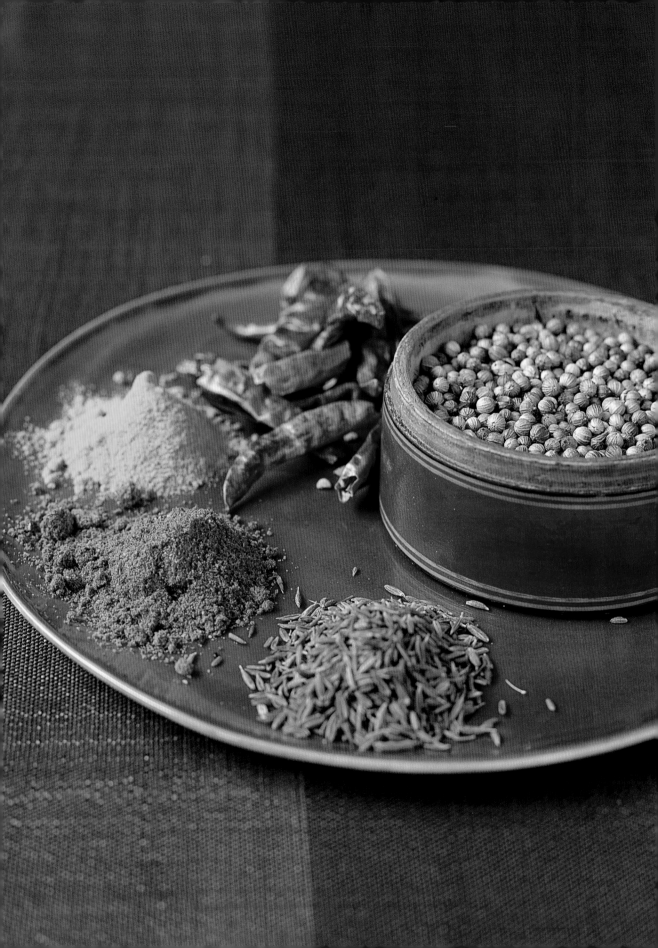

THE SPICE OF LIFE!

Sunil Vijayakar is the man behind the fantastic recipes that follow and has contributed to four previous Slimming World recipe books. He is also responsible for many of the cookery pages that appear regularly in Slimming World Magazine, helping to ensure readers stay inspired and keen to try out new dishes.

'I strongly believe that healthy food can and should taste fantastic – it's just a matter of getting good ingredients and knowing what to do with them,' says Sunil. 'For most people losing weight is a long-term process and this means that it's not a question of simply putting up with bland, boring meals for a couple of weeks and then it's all over. Long-term healthy eating, whether it's with the aim of losing weight or not, needs to be based on food that we actually enjoy eating rather than just tolerate. There is nothing about the taste of these meals that is remotely like "diet food". You could serve up any of these dishes to family and friends without them having any idea they were eating food that fitted into a healthy eating plan.'

Although Sunil is experienced in creating dishes from all over the world, working on *Slimming World's Curry Feast* was of special interest as he was born in Mumbai in India. As a young boy he used to go with his father to Sunday morning markets to buy food for that day's lunch. Together they'd wander down the aisles full of vegetables and fruit and then into open courtyards of fresh fish and shellfish, followed by stalls selling piles of nuts, spices and dried fruit.

On their return Sunil would watch his father prepare a huge lunch for family and friends with the spoils of their shopping expedition. The smells, sounds and sights – combined with the final taste of the prepared meals – left a lasting impression.

'Dad would talk to me while he was cooking about his love of different foods and ingredients and I acted as his official taster,' says Sunil. 'He was always relaxed in his attitude to preparation and cooking and most importantly he loved the gift and joy of sharing food.'

Perhaps as a direct result of this early inspiration, Sunil went on to set up a successful catering company, which he combined with working as a food stylist for the advertising and film world. He moved to London in 1993, where he lives with his wife Geraldine and their young son. He now divides his working life between

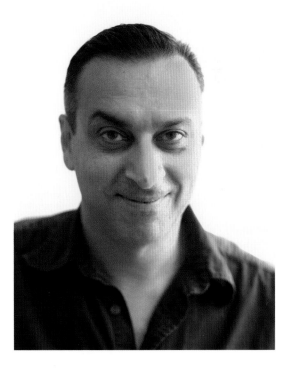

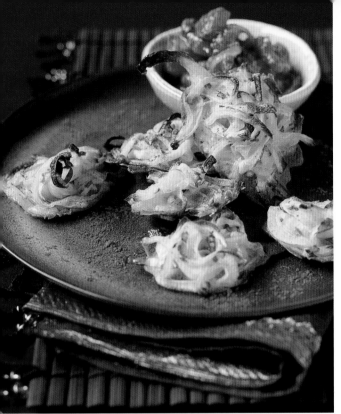
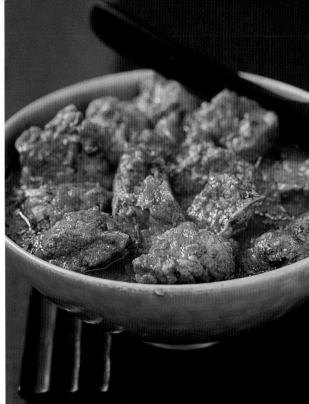

food styling and compiling recipes for numerous cookbooks – including two books on Indian food.

'Devising the recipes for this book was an interesting challenge and a lot of fun,' he says. 'The idea was to adapt a variety of dishes including the kind of popular restaurant meals we are all familiar with, such as vindaloo and jalfrezi dishes, cutting out much of the fat without affecting the flavour. I didn't know how well it was going to work with some things, like Onion bhajis (see page 52) for instance, which generally have quite a high fat content. But I was impressed with the results and the crew on the photo shoot for this book wolfed them down, so that seemed a good second opinion!

'As well as getting the best possible flavour and an authentic taste I also wanted to provide a variety of dishes to suit people's different palates, so you will see the recipes marked accordingly, but you can also adapt them to be spicier or milder depending on individual taste. The meals in this book reflect a range of different Indian traditions – from the fresh curry leaves and coconut bases of southern Indian cookery to the more robust, meat-dominated dishes of northern India. There are also a few recipes inspired by other cultures such as the Thai-style prawn and lemongrass soup and Burmese curry.'

Before you begin experimenting with the recipes, Sunil advises stocking up with a good selection of ingredients and spices. This may seem a bit expensive to start with, but a little tends to go a long way and spices will last if they are stored in airtight containers in a cool, dark place. However, Sunil warns against keeping them for too long.

'After a few months most will start to lose their flavour and not be at their best,' he says. 'As they are such an important part of this kind of cooking it is a shame to go to time and effort if the spices are old and tired so I'd recommend

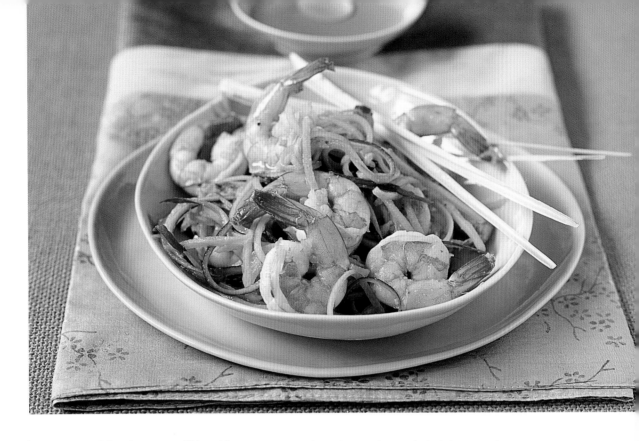

buying quantities that you will be able to use within two to three months. Hopefully you will love the recipes in this book so much that this won't be a problem because you will be getting through them!'

Most of the ingredients can be bought in large supermarkets, but Sunil's recommendation is to find an Indian or Asian greengrocer or even to order spices via the internet – he suggests trying www.seasonedpioneers.co.uk for spice blends from around the world. 'I often do this and the advantage is that they work out a lot cheaper and you can often get more in-depth advice about what you are buying,' he says.

He also recommends investing in a small coffee grinder – the type used to grind beans – for making your own curry powder. 'This is great for small quantities as you don't lose half of it up the side.' Sunil's own recipe for curry powder, which can be stored for up to a couple of months, is:

1 tbsp of coriander seeds, lightly roasted
1 tbsp of cumin seeds, lightly roasted
1 tsp turmeric
1–2 dried red chillies, crumbled
3–4 whole black peppercorns
½ tsp cardamom seeds
1–2 whole cloves
cinnamon stick (broken) or cassia bark

Grind up ingredients until they form a smooth powder, store in an airtight container and use in recipes as and when required.

FOOD OPTIMISING MENUS

Take a week or two to follow our tasty selection of mouth-watering menus and you'll be able to plan your shopping with confidence. You'll soon discover that not only does Food Optimising work, it's fabulously simple too!

These menus show the endless variety of meals that are possible when you start Food Optimising (we've included plenty of curry feasts of course!). You can be sure of plenty of nourishing, satisfying food that will keep you full and healthy – and help you lose weight too! We've included some of the recipes featured in this book.

Here's how to use Food Optimising menus most effectively:

1. Decide whether you wish to have a Green or Original day and stick to that choice all day. You can make every day a Green day or include some Original days too. Within the Green menus we have included meat-free choices suitable for vegetarians.
2. Pick one breakfast, one lunch and one dinner from your chosen set.

3. Choose around 10 to 15 Syns-worth of food from the Syns list on page 220. Some Food Optimisers find they lose weight best on 5 Syns, others on 20 Syns. On some days, you might find you perhaps need to use 30, if you are going out or celebrating. In general, we find 10 Syns a day is a good rule of thumb for effective weight loss.
4. Each day, choose twice from the following milk and cheese lists to boost your calcium intake, which is vital for a healthy diet.

MILK
* 350ml/12fl oz skimmed milk
* 225ml/8fl oz semi-skimmed milk
* 175ml/6fl oz whole milk
* 225ml/8fl oz calcium-enriched soya milk (sweetened or unsweetened)

CHEESE
* 25g/1oz Cheddar
* 25g/1oz Edam
* 25g/1oz Gouda
* 40g/1½oz Mozzarella
* 40g/1½oz reduced fat Cheddar/Cheshire
* 3 Dairylea Original triangles
* 2 mini Babybel cheeses

TIPS
* You can drink black tea and coffee, and low-calorie soft drinks, freely.
* If you want to dress your salads, fat-free French or vinaigrette-style salad dressings are Free options.

* Use artificial sweetener freely in your drinks or sprinkled over your cereals and fruit.

On the menus that are given on the following pages – divided into Green days and Original days – check out the foods that are shown in **bold**. These can be eaten freely throughout the day without any weighing or measuring. Fill up on these foods whenever you feel peckish. You can also turn to our Free Food list on page 218 and select other Free Foods to enjoy whenever you want, in whatever quantity you want.

Maximise your healthy eating by:

* Eating at least five portions of fresh fruit and vegetables every day. Frozen fruit and frozen and canned vegetables can also be used.
* Trimming any visible fat off meat and removing any skin from poultry.
* Varying your choices as much as possible to ensure the widest range of nutrients in your diet.
* Eating at least two portions of fish a week, of which one is an oily fish.
* Aiming to keep your salt intake to no more than 5g a day (1 level tsp). As well as limiting the amount of table salt you add to food, watch out for salt added to manufactured foods and sauces. Try flavouring foods with herbs and spices instead.
* Remembering the latest recommendations regarding intake of fluids, which is to aim for six to eight cups, mugs or glasses of any type of fluid per day (excluding alcohol).

Note for Slimming World members: Healthy Extra 'b' choices are built into the menus.

Once you've experienced the pleasure of Food Optimising on your plate you can design your own menus with the complete Food Optimising system, available at Slimming World groups throughout the UK.

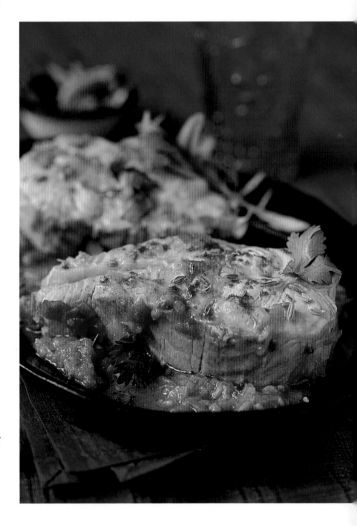

Green Menus

BREAKFASTS

1. Yogurt crunch made with **very low fat natural yogurt**, 25g/1oz Jordan's Special Muesli and sliced **kiwi** (layer the kiwi, muesli and yogurt right to the top of a tall glass finishing with a sprinkling of muesli and a slice of kiwi) followed by lots of fresh **apricots**.

2. **Quorn sausages**, any variety, grilled and served with lots of grilled **tomatoes**, **onion wedges**, poached or scrambled **eggs** and two slices of wholemeal toast, plus slices of fresh **pineapple**.

3. Fresh **grapefruit**, followed by 25g/1oz Shreddies topped with lots of **raspberries** and served with milk from your allowance, plus a pot of **Nestlé Sveltesse 0% Fat Yogurt**, any variety.

4. A large fluffy **omelette** filled with grilled **mushrooms**, **tomatoes** and 25g/1oz grated Cheddar cheese and served with plenty of **baked beans in tomato sauce**, plus a **nectarine**.

5. Chunks of **melon** topped with heaps of fresh **raspberries** followed by 25g/1oz Shredded Wheat Triple Berry served with milk from your allowance.

6. Two slices wholemeal toast topped with oodles of **baked beans in tomato sauce**, plus a bowl of chopped **pear** and **apple** smothered in **very low fat natural yogurt**.

7. Layer a pot of **Müllerlight Yogurt** with 40g/1½oz All Bran Original and frozen **berries** in a tall glass, and follow with a huge bowl of chopped **citrus fruit**.

8. 3 rashers grilled lean bacon served with lots of grilled **tomatoes** and **mushrooms**, **baked beans in tomato sauce** and a poached **egg**, plus a **peach** or two.

9. Large bowl of fresh **orange** and **grapefruit** segments followed by two Weetabix served with milk from your allowance and topped with lots of sliced **banana**.

10. Two slices wholemeal toast topped with scrambled **eggs**, followed by a bowl of fresh **strawberries** and **melon balls** topped with a **Danone Shape Solo Yogurt**, any variety.

LUNCHES

* Denotes recipe suggestion with picture.

1. 110g/4oz griddled chicken breast chunks served with **Aloo Chat** (see page 70*) and a huge crisp **salad**, followed by slices of fresh **pineapple**.

2. 50g/2oz crusty wholemeal roll filled with lots of sliced **egg**, **tomato** and mixed **salad leaves**, followed by a large bowl of fresh **strawberries**, **raspberries** and **blueberries** layered with a pot of **Danone Shape Solo Yogurt**, any variety.

3. **Mixed Vegetable Biryani** (see page 167*) followed by 350g/12oz pears canned in juice topped with plenty of **very low fat natural yogurt** flavoured with cinnamon.

4. 75g/3oz roast beef served with mountains of mashed **potatoes**, dry roast **potatoes** and **parsnips** and lots of **peas**, **carrots** and **broccoli**, followed by a 225g/8oz apple, baked and filled with 1 level tablespoon of mincemeat and topped with plenty of **very low fat natural fromage frais**.

5. **Makki-lal Mirch Bhaji** (see page 194*) served on a bed of fluffy **rice**, followed by 275g/10oz apple and 275g/10oz rhubarb stewed and topped with a **Müllerlight Vanilla Yogurt**.

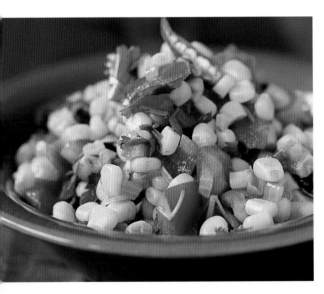

6. Large jacket **potato** filled with plenty of **baked beans in tomato sauce** and topped with 25g/1oz grated Cheddar cheese, served with a huge fresh **salad**. Plus some fresh **apricots** and **plums**.

7. 175g/6oz cod fillet/steak, grilled or poached and served with **Lemon and Turmeric Rice** (see page 164), plenty of **sweetcorn**, sugar snap peas and a large mixed **salad**. Plus a large bowl of **fresh fruit** salad made with lots of chopped **melon**, **kiwi**, **mango** and **papaya**.

8. Two slices wholemeal bread topped with 25g/1oz grated Cheddar cheese and **tomato slices** and toasted under a hot grill until the cheese bubbles, plus a pot of **Nestlé Sveltesse 0% Fat Yogurt**, any variety, and a bunch of **grapes**.

9. **Curried Carrot and Coriander Soup** (see page 48) served with a 50g/2oz crusty wholemeal roll, plus a bowl of chopped fresh **pineapple** and **peach** topped with lots of **very low fat natural yogurt** flavoured with vanilla.

10. **Pasta Salad:** mix cooked **pasta shapes** with lots of chopped **cucumber**, **tomatoes**, **beetroot**, **spring onion** and drizzle with fat-free vinaigrette. Plus lots of sliced **banana** topped with a **Müllerlight Toffee Yogurt** and sprinkled with cinnamon.

DINNERS

* Denotes recipe suggestion with picture.

1. **Khumbi Curry** (see page 199*) served with heaps of **Pea Pilau** (see page 165), followed by a bowl of fresh or frozen **summer fruits**.

2. A large **omelette** filled with chopped **peppers**, **red onions** and **sweetcorn** and served with lots of baked **potato** wedges and a large mixed **salad**. Plus half a cantaloupe **melon** piled high with **raspberries**.

3. Saag Dahi Kari (see page 202*) served with heaps of basmati **rice** and followed by a huge selection of fresh **berries** topped with spoonfuls of **very low fat natural fromage frais** flavoured with vanilla.

4. **Vegetable Stir-fry:** stir-fry lots of **broccoli** and **cauliflower** florets, chopped **carrots**, mixed **peppers**, **spring onions**, **button mushrooms**, **bean sprouts** and **water chestnuts** with a little garlic, soy sauce and some freshly chopped herbs and serve on a generous bed of **noodles**. Plus lots of **strawberries** topped with a **Müllerlight Yogurt**, any variety.

5. **Jatpatta Phool Gobi Chawal** (see page 162*), followed by a large bowl of chopped **apple**, **pear** and **grapes** topped with lots of **very low fat natural yogurt**.

6. **Quorn Lamb Grills** served with mountains of mashed **potatoes** and lots of **baby whole sweetcorn**, **carrots**, **peas** and **green beans**, plus a tropical **fresh fruit** salad made with lots of chopped **mango**, **kiwi** and **papaya**.

7. Onion Bhajis (see page 52*) followed by **Chana Masala** (see page 178*) served with plenty of shredded **cabbage** flavoured with cardamom, and white and wild **rice**, followed by **Spiced Mixed Fruit Salad** (see page 77*).

8. Large jacket **potato** topped with a can of **mixed beans** in chilli sauce and served with a generous mixed **salad**, plus a large bunch of **grapes** and a **peach** or **nectarine**.

9. Vegetable Samosas (see page 56*) followed by **Mixed Bean and Carrot Sabzi** (see page 175*), served with **Tomato and Mushroom Rice** (see page 160) plus a large bowl of **raspberries** topped with **very low fat natural fromage frais**.

10. **Tagliatelle and Mushroom Sauce:** cook some sliced **leeks**, **green pepper** and **mushrooms** in Fry Light. Pour over some **passata** and cook for 10 minutes until tender. Serve with **tagliatelle** cooked to taste. Follow with a tropical fruit skewer: push chunks of **tropical fruit** of your choice onto skewers and dip into a pot of your favourite **Müllerlight Yogurt**.

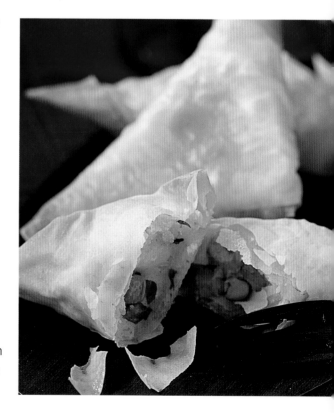

Original Menus

BREAKFASTS

1. Fresh **grapefruit** followed by lots of lean grilled **gammon**, grilled **tomatoes**, **mushrooms** and a poached **egg** served with two slices of wholemeal toast.

2. **Melon** boat filled with lots of fresh **summer fruits**, topped with **very low fat natural yogurt** and sprinkled with 25g/1oz Shredded Wheat Fruitful.

3. 250g/9oz raspberries stewed and topped with a **Müllerlight Country Berries Yogurt**, followed by plenty of grilled **kippers**, **tomatoes** and **onion** wedges.

4. Chunks of **fresh fruit** layered with a **Danone Shape Solo Yogurt**, any variety, and 40g/1½oz Alpen Crunchy Bran, plus a **banana**.

5. Two slices wholemeal toast topped with scrambled **egg** mixed with chopped **smoked salmon** and chives and served with grilled **tomatoes**, followed by a **peach** or two.

6. A large bowl of fresh **orange** and **grapefruit** segments, followed by 40g/1½oz All Bran Apricot Bites served with milk from the allowance and topped with lots of sliced **banana**.

7. Lots of grilled lean **bacon**, grilled **tomatoes**, **mushrooms**, scrambled **egg** and served with 200g/7oz new potatoes in their skins, parboiled and then sliced and fried in Fry Light. Followed by a bowl of chopped **kiwi** and **strawberries** smothered in **Nestlé Sveltesse 0% Fat Yogurt**, any variety.

8. Banana split: **banana** sliced lengthways, sprinkled with 40g/1½oz All Bran Original and topped with oodles of **very low fat natural yogurt** flavoured with cinnamon.

9. 50g/2oz wholemeal crusty roll filled with lots of grilled lean **bacon** and fresh **tomato slices**, followed by slices of fresh **pineapple**.

10. Two slices of wholemeal toast topped with lots of plum **tomatoes** with a dash of Worcestershire sauce followed by a bunch of **grapes**.

LUNCHES

* Denotes recipe suggestion with picture.

1. **Jalfrezi Chicken** (see page 128*) followed by 250g/9oz raspberries, stewed and topped with a **Danone Shape Solo Yogurt**, any variety.

2. **Dahiwalla Ghosht** (see page 100*) served with **Kachumber** (see page 212) a 225g/8oz (raw weight) jacket potato and a large crisp **salad**, followed by a huge **fresh fruit** salad of chopped **pineapple**, **peach** and **mango** smothered in **Müllerlight Yogurt**, any variety.

3. 50g/2oz wholemeal roll filled with lots of lean **ham**, sliced **tomato** and baby **salad leaves**, plus a large bunch of **grapes**.

4. **Jhinga Balti** (see page 145*) served with a 225g/8oz (raw weight) jacket potato and a huge crisp **salad**, followed by slices of fresh **pineapple**.

5. Large fluffy **omelette** filled with diced **ham** and served with lots of grilled **mushrooms**, **tomatoes** and 150g/5oz baked beans in tomato sauce followed by an **apple** and a **peach**.

6. **Lemongrass Prawn Salad** (see page 80*) followed by **Saag Walla Turkey** (see page 134*) served with lots of **Sukki Gobi** (see page 192), plus 350g/12oz apricots canned in juice.

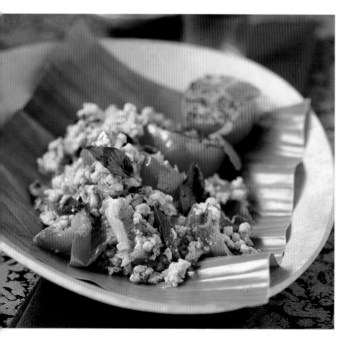

7. **Kheema with Curry Leaves** (see page 90*) with **Garam Masala Tamater** (see page 187) and served with a 50g/2oz crusty wholemeal roll, followed by a large bowl of **strawberries** topped with lashings of **very low fat natural yogurt**.

8. A large grilled **chicken breast** served with 200g/7oz new potatoes in their skins and plenty of **asparagus**, **carrots** and **broccoli**, followed by lots of chopped **apple** and **pear** topped with oodles of **very low fat natural fromage frais** flavoured with vanilla.

9. BLT: two slices wholemeal bread filled with lots of grilled **bacon**, **tomato slices** and crisp **salad leaves**, followed by a bowl of chopped **melon**, **kiwi** and **strawberries**.

10. Lots of roast **lamb** served with mint sauce, 200g/7oz new potatoes in their skins and plenty of **cabbage**, **carrots**, **baby whole sweetcorn** and **green beans**, followed by a **fresh fruit salad** smothered in **Nestlé Sveltesse 0% Fat Yogurt**, any variety.

DINNERS
* Denotes recipe suggestion with picture.

1. **Masala Crab Cakes** (see page 61*) followed by **Pork Vindaloo** (see page 95*) served with lots of steamed **courgettes** and **carrots**, plus lots of sliced **banana** smothered in **Müllerlight Toffee Yogurt**.

2. **Melon** boat piled high with **strawberries** followed by **Shahi Murgh** (see page 123*) served with Naryal Chutney (see page 216*) and lots of **broccoli** and **cauliflower** florets and **green beans**.

3. **Salmon fillet**, cooked with Cajun spices, served with heaps of **asparagus**, **mangetout**, and **baby whole sweetcorn**, followed by a **peach** and a few **plums**.

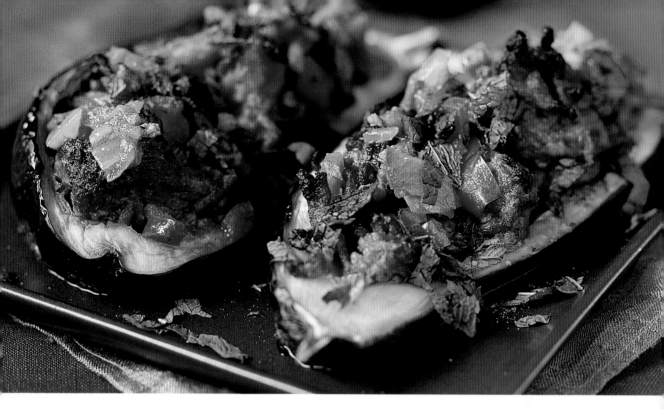

4. **Stuffed Aubergines with Spiced Lamb** (see page 104*) served with **Mooli Gajjar Raita** (see page 207) and plenty of **cabbage** flavoured with cardamom, followed with slices of **honeydew melon**.

5. Lean **gammon** steak, grilled, topped with fresh **pineapple** slices and served with a plateful of **salad leaves, cherry tomatoes, cucumber, spring onions** and grated **carrot**. Followed by **peaches** or **nectarines**.

6. **Beef Kofta Curry** (see page 108*) served with heaps of **green beans** and **baby whole sweetcorn**, followed by lots of fresh chopped **mango** and sliced **grapes** topped with oodles of **very low fat natural yogurt**.

7. **Citrus Pork & Lettuce Salad** (see page 86*) followed by **Kerala Style Fish in Banana Leaves** (see page 153*) served with lots of

Curried Butternut Squash (see page 186). Plus a large bowl of chopped **pineapple, kiwi, melon** and **strawberries**.

8. **Classic Chicken Curry** (see page 116*) served with plenty of **carrots, sugar snap peas** and **cauliflower**, followed by a large bowl of **summerfruits** smothered in **Nestlé Sveltesse 0% Fat Yogurt**, any variety.

9. Lots of lean roast **beef** served with heaps of **baby whole sweetcorn, green beans, broccoli** and mashed **swede**, followed by a large bowl of **raspberries, blackberries** and **blueberries** topped with **very low fat natural fromage frais**.

10. A lean boneless **pork** steak, grilled or baked, served with lots of oven roasted vegetables: chunks of **red, yellow** and **green pepper, red onion** wedges, **tomato** halves, and a large **green salad**, followed by slices of fresh **pineapple**.

SYN-FREE STORECUPBOARD

All these storecupboard ingredients are Free Foods for both Green and Original days, unless otherwise stated.

CANS AND BOTTLES

Artificial sweetener
Baked beans in tomato sauce (Green days)
Black-eye beans (Green days)
Butter beans (Green days)
Chickpeas (Green days)
Fat-free dressings, French-style & vinaigrette
Green peppercorns in brine
Red kidney beans (Green days)
Lean canned ham (Original days)
Mixed beans (Green days)
Sweetcorn (Green days)
Tomatoes, plum and chopped

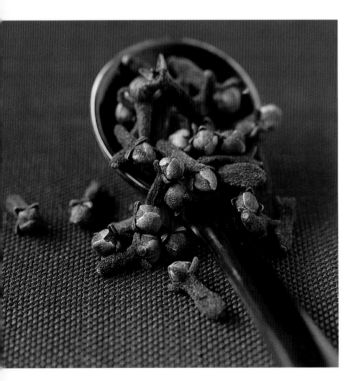

FROM THE FRIDGE

Chillies, red and green
Fresh herbs, e.g.
    bay leaf
    coriander
    curry leaves
    kaffir lime leaves
    lemongrass
    mint
    parsley (standard and flat-leaf)
Ginger, fresh root
Spring onions
Very low fat natural fromage frais
Very low fat natural yogurt

STAPLES

Bovril stock, all varieties
Dried bay leaves
Dried red chillies
Fry Light
Galangal (type of ginger)
Lentils, all varieties (Green days)
Mixed dried herbs: all varieties
Mustard, powdered
Nam pla (fish sauce)
Passata
Pasta, all types, dried (Green days)
Rice: all varieties, e.g. Basmati, long grain, brown, wild (Green days)
Soy sauces, dark and light
Spice rack of ground and whole spices, e.g.
    amchoor (dried mango powder)
    black and mixed peppercorns
    black onion seeds (nigella)
    cardamom (pods and seeds)
    cayenne

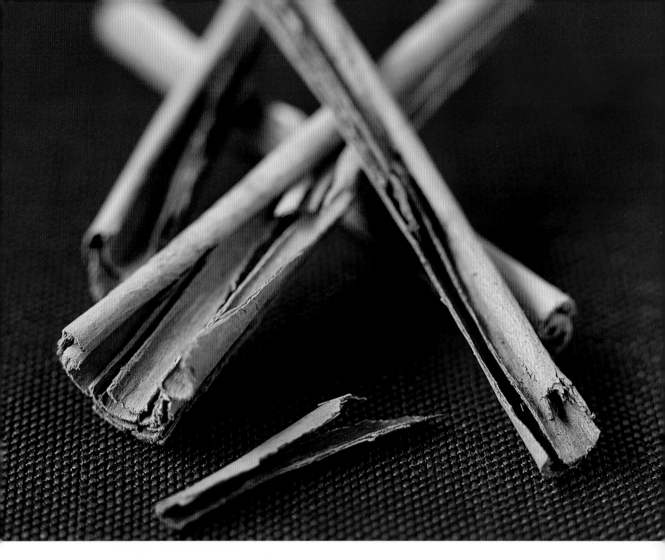

chilli powder (mild, medium and hot)
cinnamon (ground and sticks)
cloves
coriander (ground and seeds)
cumin (ground and seeds)
curry powder (a range of different varieties from mild to hot, e.g. madras, korma, tikka masala)
fennel seeds
fenugreek seeds
garam masala
ground cardamom
ground ginger
mustard seeds (black and yellow)
nutmeg
paprika

sea salt
tandoori spice blend
turmeric
Tabasco sauce
Vecon
Vinegars: e.g. malt, white, white wine

ON THE KITCHEN WORKTOP

Eggs
Garlic
Lemons and limes
Onions and shallots
Tomatoes, all kinds

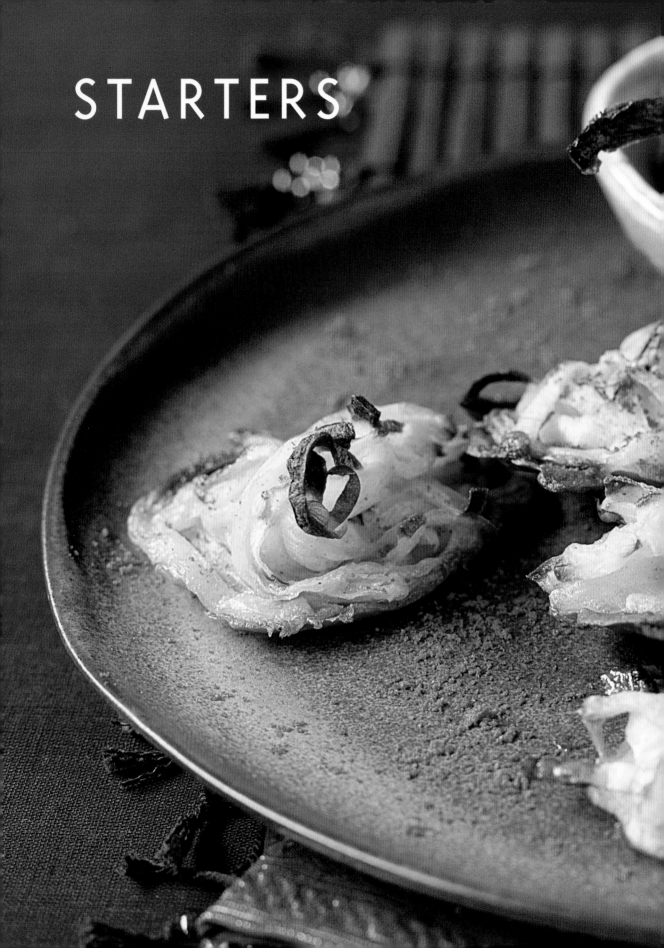

STARTERS

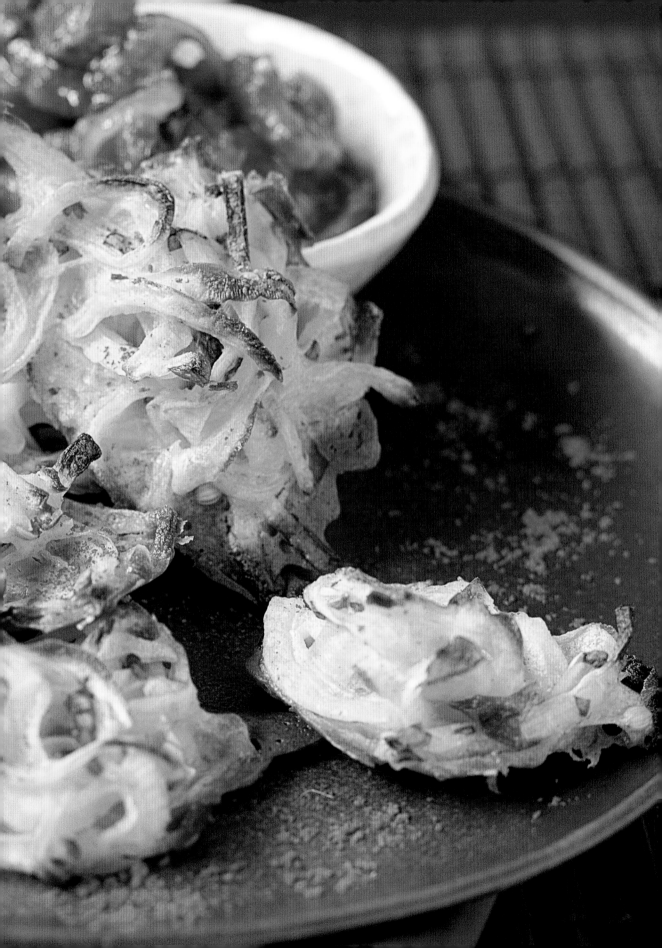

THAI GREEN CURRY SOUP

MEDIUM 🌶🌶

A rich and aromatic soup made from fresh chicken breasts flavoured with lemon-grass, lime leaves, galangal (a type of ginger) and creamy coconut milk.

SERVES 4 ❄
Syns per serving
Original: 1
EASY
Preparation time 5 minutes
Cooking time 40 minutes

2 chicken breasts, skinless and boneless

4 kaffir lime leaves, finely shredded

2 tbsp very finely chopped lemongrass stalks

1 tsp very finely grated galangal

1.25 litres/2 pints chicken stock made with Bovril

juice of 1 lime

6 tbsp very finely chopped coriander leaves

2 tsp nam pla

1 fresh red chilli, deseeded and very finely sliced

4 tbsp reduced-fat coconut milk

4 spring onions, trimmed and very finely sliced

salt and freshly ground black pepper

1. Place the chicken, kaffir lime leaves, lemongrass, galangal and chicken stock in a medium saucepan and bring to the boil.

2. Reduce the heat to low, cover and simmer gently for 20–25 minutes or until the chicken is cooked through. Using a slotted spoon, remove the chicken from the saucepan and, using your fingers, tear the flesh into bite-sized shreds.

3. Return the chicken to the saucepan with the lime juice, coriander leaves, nam pla, red chilli, coconut milk and most of the spring onions. Season well and heat gently for 4–5 minutes until warmed through. Serve immediately in warmed bowls, garnished with the remaining spring onion.

TIP Don't worry if you can't find all of the ingredients in your local supermarket. The kaffir lime leaves can be swapped for the zest of two limes; the grated galangal can be replaced with root ginger; and the nam pla can be substituted with light soy sauce.

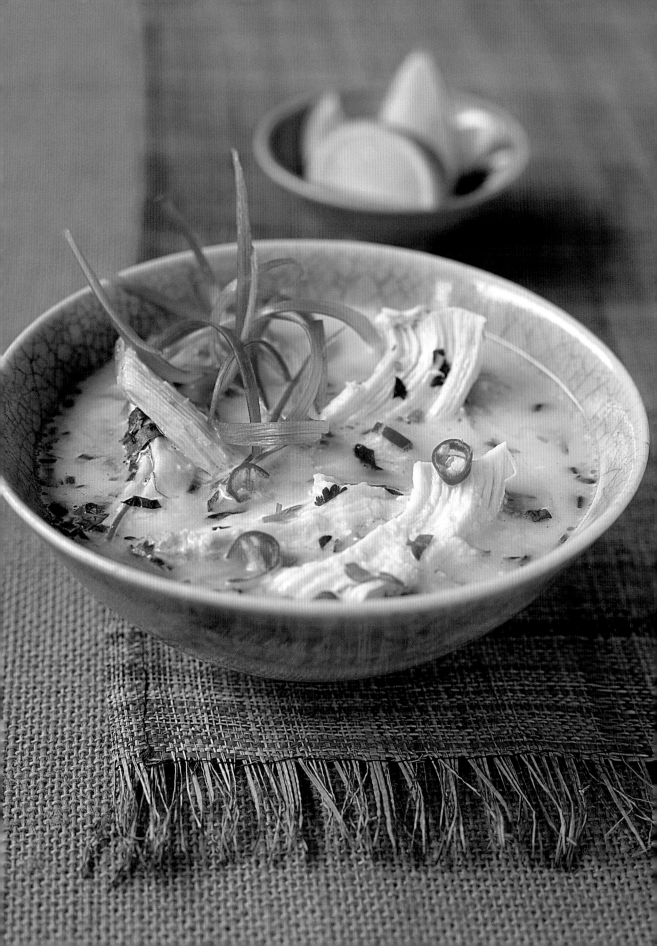

CURRIED CARROT AND CORIANDER SOUP

MILD 🌶

This warming soup is gently spiced with cumin, cardamom and coriander and is also delicious served chilled on a hot summer's day.

SERVES 4 Ⓥ ❄
Syns per serving
Green: Free
Original: Free

EASY
Preparation time 10 minutes
Cooking time 50 minutes

Fry Light

1 onion, peeled and finely chopped

1 tsp ground cumin

½ tsp ground coriander

¼ tsp mild chilli powder

¼ tsp crushed cardamom seeds

2 garlic cloves, peeled and crushed

600g/1lb 6oz carrots, peeled and roughly chopped

salt and freshly ground black pepper

8 tbsp finely chopped coriander leaves

TO SERVE
4 tbsp very low fat natural yogurt

1. Spray a large non-stick saucepan with Fry Light and place over a medium heat. Add the onion and fry for 4–5 minutes until softened. Add the ground spices and garlic and continue to stir-fry for 1–2 minutes.

2. Add the carrots and 800ml/28fl oz of water. Bring to the boil, cover and then simmer gently for 25–30 minutes or until the carrots are tender. Season well, allow to cool slightly then place in a food processor and blend until smooth.

3. Return the soup to the saucepan and reheat gently. Ladle into four warmed bowls, stir in the chopped coriander and top each serving with a tablespoon of yogurt.

SPICY CUMIN AND
PUMPKIN SOUP

MILD ✐

This warming, lightly spiced soup marries the flavours of pumpkin with cumin to produce a soup that is deliciously comforting. To ring a change, replace the pumpkin with butternut squash.

SERVES 4 Ⓥ ❄
Syns per serving
Green: Free
Original: Free

WORTH THE EFFORT
Preparation time 10 minutes
Cooking time 35 minutes

Fry Light

1 onion, peeled and finely chopped

1.2kg/2lb 11oz pumpkin, peeled, deseeded and roughly chopped

1 tbsp ground cumin

salt and freshly ground black pepper

750ml/26fl oz vegetable stock made with Vecon

2 tbsp finely chopped coriander leaves

TO SERVE

4 tbsp very low fat natural yogurt

roasted cumin seeds

paprika

1. Spray a non-stick saucepan with Fry Light and place over a medium heat. Add the chopped onion to the pan and stir-fry for 3–4 minutes until softened.

2. Add the pumpkin and ground cumin and stir-fry for 2–3 minutes. Season well, add the stock and bring to the boil. Cover, lower the heat and simmer gently for 20–25 minutes or until the pumpkin is tender.

3. Allow the soup to cool slightly, place in a food processor and blend until smooth. Stir in the coriander and ladle the soup into warmed bowls. Garnish each bowl with a spoonful of yogurt and a sprinkling of roasted cumin seeds and paprika.

CHILLED SPINACH AND YOGURT SOUP

Originally made with buttermilk, this refreshing chilled soup is a treat on a warm summer's day.

SERVES 4 Ⓥ
Syns per serving
Green: Free
Original: Free

EXTRA EASY
Preparation time 10 minutes
Cooking time none

250g/9oz frozen baby spinach leaves, defrosted

1 garlic clove, peeled and crushed

½ tsp peeled and finely grated ginger

500g pot very low fat natural yogurt

salt and freshly ground black pepper

3 tsp dried mint

TO SERVE
freshly chopped mint leaves

1. Squeeze the water from the spinach and chop very finely. Place in a large mixing bowl with the garlic, ginger and yogurt. Season well and stir in the dried mint.

2. Add 350ml/12fl oz of really cold water and briefly process the mixture in a blender until smooth.

3. To serve, ladle into chilled bowls with a couple of cubes of ice in each one and garnish with a few fresh mint leaves.

QUAIL EGGS WITH SPICED SALT

MEDIUM

Spiced salt mixtures are used in India to dip raw vegetables and sometimes fruit into as a snack. Here we use boiled quail eggs as a dipper for this delicious and easy starter.

SERVES 4 ⓥ
Syns per serving
Green: Free
Original: Free

EXTRA EASY
Preparation time 5 minutes
Cooking time 10 minutes

24 fresh quail eggs

4 tbsp sea salt

1 tsp mild or medium coarse chilli powder

1 tbsp roasted coriander seeds, lightly crushed

1 tbsp roasted cumin seeds, lightly crushed

1 tbsp roasted fennel seeds, lightly crushed

1. Place the eggs in a saucepan of cold water and bring to the boil. Reduce the heat and allow to simmer gently for 5–6 minutes.

2. Drain and immerse in cold water. Peel the eggs carefully and place on a serving platter to cool.

3. Meanwhile, mix together the remaining ingredients and place in a small dipping bowl. Serve the quail eggs and allow your guests to dip them into the salt mixture.

TIP You can make the spiced salt and store it in an airtight container or jar for up to one month.

ONION BHAJIS

These classic bhajis are delicious served hot with Khatta-meetta tamatar chutney (see page 213).

MAKES 12 Ⓥ ❄

Syns per serving
Green: 1
Original: 1

WORTH THE EFFORT
Preparation time 10 minutes
(plus resting)
Cooking time 20 minutes

200g/7oz onions, peeled, halved and thinly sliced

50g/2oz gram flour

1 tsp lemon juice

2 tsp ground cumin

1 tbsp coriander seeds, crushed

1 tsp deseeded and chopped fresh green chilli

1 tbsp freshly chopped coriander leaves

¼ tsp baking powder

salt

Fry Light

TO SERVE
a pinch of paprika

1. Place the onions, gram flour, lemon juice, cumin, coriander seeds, green chilli, chopped coriander and baking powder in a mixing bowl. Season with salt and add a few tablespoons of water to form a thick batter that coats the onion. Leave to rest for 15 minutes and then, using your fingers, mix again to combine thoroughly.

2. Preheat the oven to 220°C/Gas 7. Line a baking sheet with baking parchment and using your fingers or a dessert spoon, drop small mounds of the mixture onto the prepared baking sheet to give you 12 bhajis.

3. Spray with Fry Light and bake for 15–20 minutes until golden. Remove from the oven and serve immediately sprinkled with the paprika.

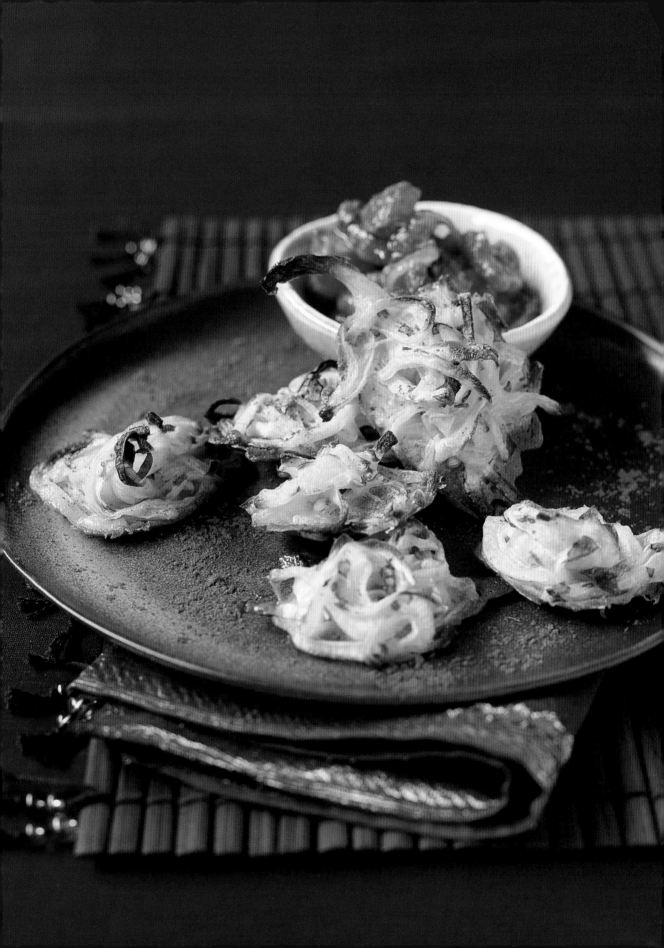

MUSHROOM BHAJIS

MEDIUM

These spiced mushroom fritters are baked rather than deep fried. In India, all sorts of vegetables, like aubergine, cauliflower florets, potato slices and onions, are used in making bhajis. They are a classic snack or street-food speciality. Here they are wonderful as a starter when served with a crisp green salad.

SERVES 4 Ⓥ ❄
Syns per serving
Green: 2½
Original: 2½

EASY
Preparation time 10 minutes
Cooking time 20 minutes

50g/2oz gram flour
1 tbsp ground coriander
1 tbsp ground cumin
1 tsp mild or medium chilli powder
2 tsp sea salt
½ tsp baking powder
1 tsp fennel seeds
12 large mushrooms, halved
Fry Light
chopped coriander leaves

TO SERVE
crisp green salad

1. Preheat the oven to 220°C/Gas 7. In a mixing bowl, combine the gram flour, ground coriander, ground cumin, chilli powder, sea salt, baking powder and fennel seeds.

2. Add 2 tablespoons of cold water to make a thick batter.

3. Coat the mushrooms in the batter and place on a baking tray lined with baking parchment. Spray with Fry Light and bake in the oven for 15–20 minutes or until lightly golden. Remove from the oven, sprinkle over the chopped coriander and serve immediately with a crisp green salad.

TIP Use bite-sized cauliflower florets as an alternative. Coat them with the batter and bake until tender.

CHICKPEA PATTIES

MILD ✦

This street-food snack of spicy chickpea and potato cakes can be found through-out the length and breadth of India. Usually fried, here they are baked for a healthy, delicious starter.

SERVES 4 Ⓥ ❋
Syns per serving
Green: Free
WORTH THE EFFORT
Preparation time 20 minutes
(plus chilling)
Cooking time 30 minutes

400g can chickpeas, drained

1 onion, peeled and very finely chopped

200g/7oz freshly mashed potato

2 tsp mild chilli powder

¼ tsp turmeric

1 small egg, lightly beaten

1 tsp roasted coriander seeds, crushed

2 tsp roasted cumin seeds, crushed

2 tbsp finely chopped mint leaves

2 tbsp finely chopped coriander leaves

salt

Fry Light

1. Place the chickpeas and onion in a food processor and blend for 1–2 minutes or until roughly mashed. Transfer to a mixing bowl and add the potatoes, chilli powder, turmeric, egg, roasted coriander and cumin seeds and the chopped herbs. Season well with salt, cover and chill in the fridge for 5–6 hours or overnight.

2. Preheat the oven to 200°C/Gas 6. Divide the chickpea mixture into 12 portions and shape each one into a flat cake or patty.

3. Place the patties on a baking tray lined with baking parchment. Spray with Fry Light and bake for 20–25 minutes or until lightly golden and cooked through. Serve immediately with Cucumber, chilli and mint raita (see page 211) or Hara chutney (see page 210).

VEGETABLE SAMOSAS

These crispy vegetable filled pastries are a classic Indian favourite. Traditionally deep fried, here they are lightly sprayed with Fry Light and then baked to give you a delicious and healthy version.

MAKES 18 Ⓥ ❄

Syns per serving
Green: 1
Original: 2

WORTH THE EFFORT
Preparation time 30 minutes
Cooking time 20 minutes

Fry Light

1 tbsp mild curry powder

1 tsp amchoor (dried mango powder)

400g/14oz potatoes, peeled, boiled and mashed

110g/4oz fresh or frozen peas

4 tbsp finely chopped coriander leaves

1 fresh red chilli, deseeded and finely chopped

salt

3 large sheets filo pastry

1. Spray a large non-stick frying pan with Fry Light and place over a medium heat. Add the curry powder, amchoor, potatoes and peas and stir-fry for 4–5 minutes. Remove from the heat and add the coriander leaves and chilli, season well with salt and set aside.

2. Preheat the oven to 190°C/Gas 5. Line a large baking sheet with baking parchment. Working swiftly, place the three filo sheets on top of each other and cut them in half widthways. Then cut each half into three even strips lengthways to give you a total of six strips of filo per sheet (18 strips in total).

3. Lay the strips on a clean work surface and lightly spray with Fry Light. Place a teaspoonful of the potato filling at the bottom of each strip and fold the pastry diagonally to enclose the filling and form a triangle. Press down on the pastry and fold again until you reach the end of the strip, leaving you with a triangular pastry parcel. Repeat with the remaining strips and filling to make 18 parcels.

4. Place the parcels in a single layer on the prepared baking sheet, spray with Fry Light and bake for 15–20 minutes or until golden and crisp. Remove from the oven and serve warm with the Hara chutney (see page 210).

WHAT IS IT? In Hindi, *amchoor* translates simply as 'mango powder'. The mango is picked before it ripens, peeled and cut into thin slices and sun dried. This is then ground into a powder. It is used to give a tangy flavour to Indian recipes. You can buy it from large supermarkets and Asian greengrocers.

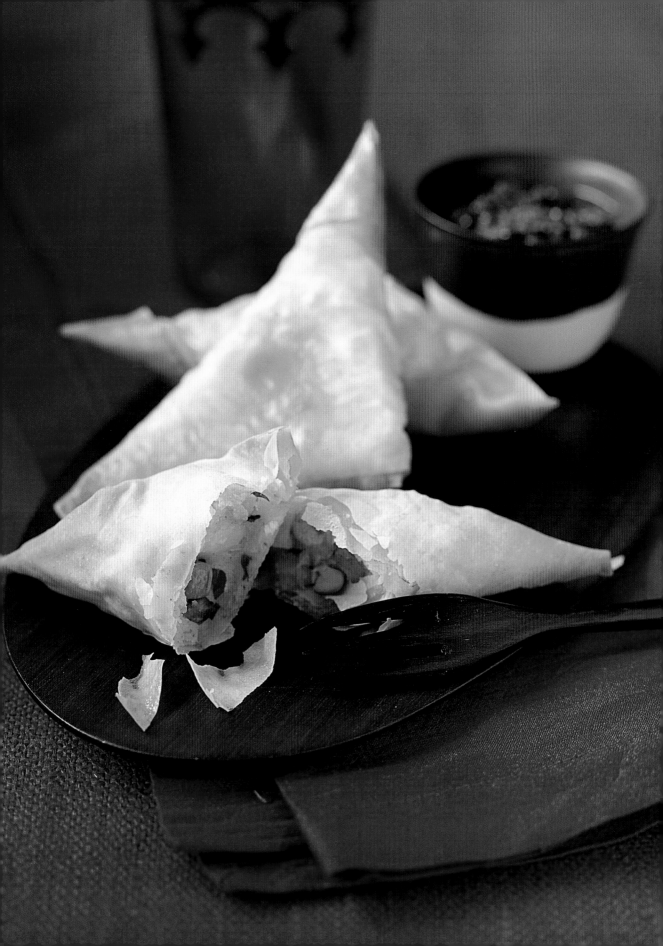

MARINE DRIVE BHUTA

MEDIUM 🌶🌶

Along the seafront in Mumbai on Marine Drive, there are street vendors with little barbecues grilling fresh corn-on-the-cob. They are then quickly rubbed with a chilli, lime and salt mixture and served on the corn husks ... which makes this a really easy and memorable starter!

SERVES 4 ⓥ
Syns per serving
Green: Free

EXTRA EASY
Preparation time 5 minutes
Cooking time 10 minutes

4 fresh corn-on-the-cob
2 tbsp sea salt
2 tsp mild or medium coarse chilli powder
2 limes, halved

1. Strip the husks from the corn and reserve to serve the finished dish on. Hold the corn under cold running water to remove the silken threads.

2. Mix the sea salt and chilli powder in a small bowl and set aside.

3. Over a barbecue or under a hot grill, cook the corn for 6–8 minutes, turning often to cook evenly, until the corn is lightly charred in a few places and cooked through.

4. Remove the corn from the heat and dip the cut side of a lime half in the salt and chilli mixture and use to rub into the cooked corn, squeezing the juice of the lime onto it. Repeat with the remaining corn and lime and serve immediately on the husks of corn.

TOFU AND MANGO KEBABS MEDIUM ♪♪

Tofu is used as a low fat substitute for the Indian cheese 'paneer' in this delicious starter that is quick and easy to prepare.

SERVES 4 Ⓥ
Syns per serving
Green: 2
Original: 2

EASY
Preparation time 30 minutes
(plus marinating)
Cooking time 10 minutes

500g/1lb 2oz firm tofu

1 large mango, peeled, stoned and cubed

FOR THE MARINADE

2 fresh red chillies, deseeded and chopped

2 garlic cloves, peeled and crushed

1 tbsp peeled and finely grated ginger

1 tbsp clear honey

finely grated zest and juice of 1 lime

salt

1. Cover a chopping board with several layers of kitchen paper and place the tofu on top. Cover with more kitchen paper, place another board on top, weigh down with a can of beans and allow the tofu to drain for about 30 minutes. Remove the tofu from the board and cut into 2.5cm/1in cubes.

2. Meanwhile, make the marinade by combining all the ingredients in a shallow bowl. Add the tofu cubes and toss well to coat evenly. Allow to marinate for 20–30 minutes.

3. Lift the tofu out of the marinade and thread onto eight skewers alternately with the mango cubes. Grill the kebabs under a medium-hot grill for 6–8 minutes, turning them once or twice until the tofu is lightly browned and heated through. Serve immediately.

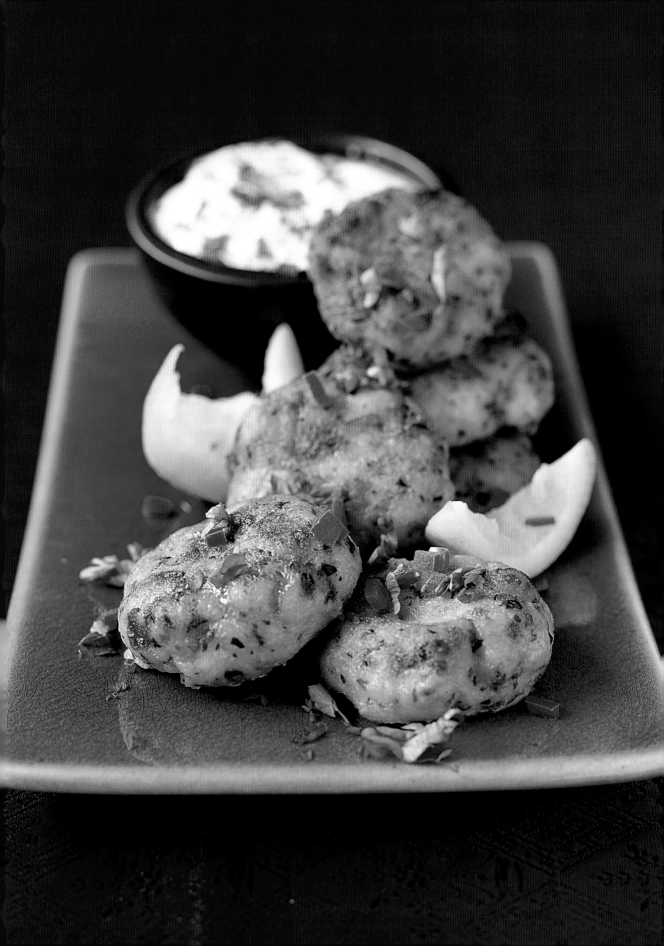

MASALA CRAB CAKES

These crab cakes originate from the southern coast of western India and here they are mixed with a firm white fish to give a spicy, flavoursome cake that is a great starter or could make a terrific light lunch when served with a salad.

SERVES 4 ❄️
Syns per serving
Original: Free

EASY
Preparation time 5 minutes
(plus chilling)
Cooking time 25 minutes

200g/7oz fresh white crabmeat

200g/7oz white fish fillet (cod or halibut), roughly chopped

1 tbsp mild curry powder

2 garlic cloves, peeled and crushed

1 fresh red chilli, deseeded and finely chopped

4 tbsp peeled and finely chopped red onion

4 tbsp freshly chopped coriander leaves, plus a little to garnish

1 small egg, beaten

salt and freshly ground black pepper

Fry Light

TO SERVE
finely chopped red pepper

lemon wedges

very low fat natural yogurt

1. Place the crabmeat, white fish, curry powder, garlic, red chilli, red onion, coriander and egg in a food processor. Season well and blend for a few seconds until well mixed. Transfer to a mixing bowl and, using your fingers, mix well. Cover and chill in the fridge for 5–6 hours (or overnight if possible) to allow the mixture to firm up and let the flavours combine.

2. Preheat the oven to 200°C/Gas 6. Line a baking sheet with non-stick baking parchment and spray with Fry Light. Divide the crab mixture into 12 portions and shape each one into a 'cake'.

3. Place on the prepared baking sheet and bake for 20–25 minutes or until lightly browned and cooked through. Serve immediately garnished with coriander, red pepper and lemon wedges, with the yogurt on the side to dip into.

GINGER CHICKEN WINGS

Adrakh or fresh root ginger is widely used in Indian cuisine to impart a rich flavour to many vegetable, meat and poultry dishes. In this recipe it is used to add extra flavour to chicken wings.

SERVES 4 ❄

Syns per serving
Original: Free

EXTRA EASY
Preparation time 5 minutes
(plus marinating)
Cooking time 15 minutes

12 large chicken wings, skinless

2 tsp peeled and finely grated ginger

2 tsp sea salt

2 tsp Tabasco sauce

2 garlic cloves, peeled and crushed

juice of 2 lemons

½ tsp artificial sweetener

4 tbsp very low fat natural yogurt

Fry Light

TO SERVE
mixed salad leaves

1. Place the chicken wings in a large mixing bowl. Mix together the ginger, sea salt, Tabasco, garlic, lemon juice, sweetener and yogurt and pour over the chicken. Toss well to combine, cover and marinate in the fridge overnight.

2. When ready to cook, remove the wings from the marinade, place on a grill rack and lightly spray with Fry Light.

3. Cook under a medium grill for 10–12 minutes, turning once or twice or until they are cooked through and lightly browned. Serve immediately on a bed of mixed salad leaves.

HARA KEBABS

These spiced Indian green chicken kebabs are a northern Indian speciality and can be a wonderful addition to any summer's day barbecue.

SERVES 4 ❄

Syns per serving
Original: Free

EASY

Preparation time 10 minutes
(plus marinating)

Cooking time 10 minutes

4 chicken breasts, skinless and boneless, cut into bite-sized pieces

juice of 1 lime

6 tbsp very low fat natural yogurt

1 tsp peeled and finely grated ginger

1 garlic clove, peeled and crushed

1 fresh green chilli, deseeded and chopped

a small handful of chopped coriander leaves

a small handful of chopped mint leaves

½ tsp ground cumin

1 tsp ground coriander

¼ tsp turmeric

salt

TO SERVE
lime wedges

1. Place the chicken pieces in a large bowl and then put the remaining ingredients in a food processor and blend until fairly smooth, adding a little water if necessary. Pour over the chicken and toss to mix well. Cover and leave to marinate in the fridge overnight.

2. To cook, thread the chicken onto eight metal skewers and place under a hot grill or on a barbecue and cook for 6–8 minutes, turning once or twice until the chicken is cooked through. Serve immediately with wedges of lime.

TANDOORI LAMB CHOPS

Tandoors are traditional clay ovens used for cooking meat, fish and breads in northern India. Here the marinated lamb chops are cooked in an oven. The chops used in this recipe are a particularly lean cut of lamb available from large supermarkets or ask your local butcher.

SERVES 4 ❋
Syns per serving
Original: ½

EASY
Preparation time 5 minutes
(plus marinating)
Cooking time 15 minutes

12 lamb chops from a French trimmed rack of lamb

4 tbsp very low fat natural yogurt

2 tbsp tomato purée

2 tsp ground coriander

1 tsp peeled and finely grated ginger

1 tsp hot chilli powder

2 tsp sea salt

3 tbsp lemon juice

Fry Light

TO SERVE
red onion rings
tomato slices
cucumber slices

1. Place the chops in a single layer in a shallow dish.

2. In a small bowl mix together the yogurt, tomato purée, ground coriander, ginger, chilli powder, sea salt and lemon juice and rub into the lamb. Cover and marinate for 4–5 hours or overnight if time permits.

3. Preheat the oven to 220°C/Gas 7. Spread the lamb chops in a single layer on a baking sheet that has been lined with baking parchment. Lightly spray with Fry Light and place in the oven for 12–15 minutes or until the lamb is cooked to your liking. Remove and serve immediately with the red onion rings, tomato and cucumber slices.

SEEKH KEBABS

MEDIUM ⁊⁊

These aromatic and spiced minced beef kebabs are often cooked on open braziers or grills in small roadside restaurants throughout northern India. Here they are baked to perfection and make a great starter.

SERVES 4 ❄

Syns per serving
Original: Free

EASY

Preparation time 15 minutes
(plus marinating)

Cooking time 20 minutes

1 fresh green chilli, deseeded and finely chopped

2 tsp ground ginger

5 garlic cloves, peeled and crushed

2 tbsp finely chopped coriander leaves

1 tsp roasted cumin seeds

500g/1lb 2oz extra-lean minced beef

2 tbsp peeled and very finely chopped red onion

1 tsp mild or medium chilli powder

1 small egg, beaten

2 tsp sea salt

Fry Light

TO SERVE
lemon wedges

1. Place all the ingredients (except the Fry Light and lemon wedges) in a mixing bowl and use your fingers to combine thoroughly. Cover and marinate in the fridge overnight to allow the flavours to develop.

2. Preheat the oven to 190°C/Gas 5 and line a baking sheet with baking parchment. Divide the meat mixture into 12 portions and shape each one around a metal or bamboo skewer to make a sausage shape about 10cm/4in in length.

3. Place the kebabs on the prepared baking sheet and lightly spray with Fry Light. Bake for 15–20 minutes, turning them once halfway through cooking. Remove from the oven and serve immediately with wedges of lemon to squeeze over.

SALADS

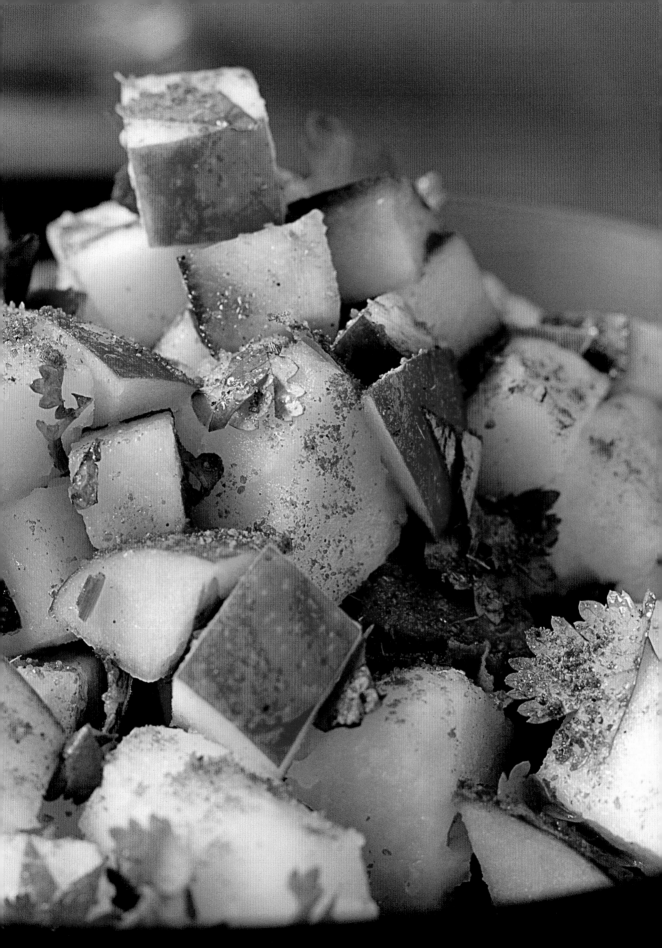

BABY SPINACH AND COCONUT SALAD

MILD 🌶

Coconuts are widely used in southern Indian coastal cooking. In this recipe they are teamed with baby spinach to give you a refreshing and tasty salad.

SERVES 4 Ⓥ
Syns per serving
Green: 1½
Original: 1½

EASY
Preparation time 10 minutes
Cooking time 1 minute

300g/11oz fresh baby spinach leaves, finely chopped

1 small carrot, peeled and coarsely grated

25g/1oz fresh coconut, grated

Fry Light

1 tsp black mustard seeds

1 tsp cumin seeds

juice of 1 lime

salt and freshly ground black pepper

1. Place the spinach in a large mixing bowl along with the grated carrot and coconut.

2. Heat a frying pan sprayed with Fry Light. Add the mustard and cumin seeds and stir-fry for 20–30 seconds.

3. Remove from the heat and add to the salad mixture along with the lime juice. Season to taste and toss well before serving.

MOOLI SALAD

Mooli or white radish makes a refreshing salad and is the perfect accompaniment to any meal. It is now available in larger supermarkets or commonly available at Asian greengrocers.

SERVES 4 Ⓥ
Syns per serving
Green: Free
Original: Free

EASY
Preparation time 10 minutes
(plus chilling)
Cooking time none

150g pot very low fat natural
fromage frais

salt and freshly ground black
pepper

¼ tsp ground cumin

1 tbsp finely chopped mint
leaves

1 small red onion, peeled and
very finely sliced

450g/1lb mooli or white radish

1. Beat the fromage frais in a bowl until smooth and season well with salt and black pepper. Stir in the cumin, mint and red onion and mix well.

2. Peel the mooli using a vegetable peeler and coarsely grate into a large mixing bowl.

3. Add the fromage frais mixture to it and toss to mix well. Cover and chill until you are ready to serve the salad.

TIP If mooli is unavailable, use the same quantity of finely sliced red radish instead.

ALOO CHAT

MEDIUM

Aloo is the Indian word for potatoes and chat is the name given to any fruit or vegetable salad spiced with 'chat masala'. Chat masala can be made and stored in an airtight container for up to a month.

SERVES 4 Ⓥ
Syns per serving
Green: Free

EASY
Preparation time 20 minutes
(plus chilling)
Cooking time none

FOR THE CHAT MASALA

1 tbsp freshly ground black pepper

2 tbsp sea salt

1 tbsp dry-roasted cumin seeds, roughly ground

3 tsp amchoor (dried mango powder)

1 tsp mild or medium coarse red chilli powder

FOR THE ALOO

1 red apple, cored and cut into small cubes

3 potatoes, boiled and cut into small cubes

1 small cucumber, cut into small cubes

juice of 1 lemon

4 tsp chat masala

a handful of freshly chopped coriander and mint leaves

1. Mix together all the ingredients for the chat masala and store in an airtight container until needed.

2. For the aloo, place the apple, potatoes, cucumber and lemon juice in a mixing bowl and sprinkle over the chat masala. Toss to mix well and cover and chill in the fridge for 30 minutes to allow the flavours and the spices to develop.

3. Just before serving, toss in the herbs and mix well. Serve immediately.

TIP If you don't have time to make your own chat masala, you can always buy it ready prepared from large supermarkets and Asian greengrocers.

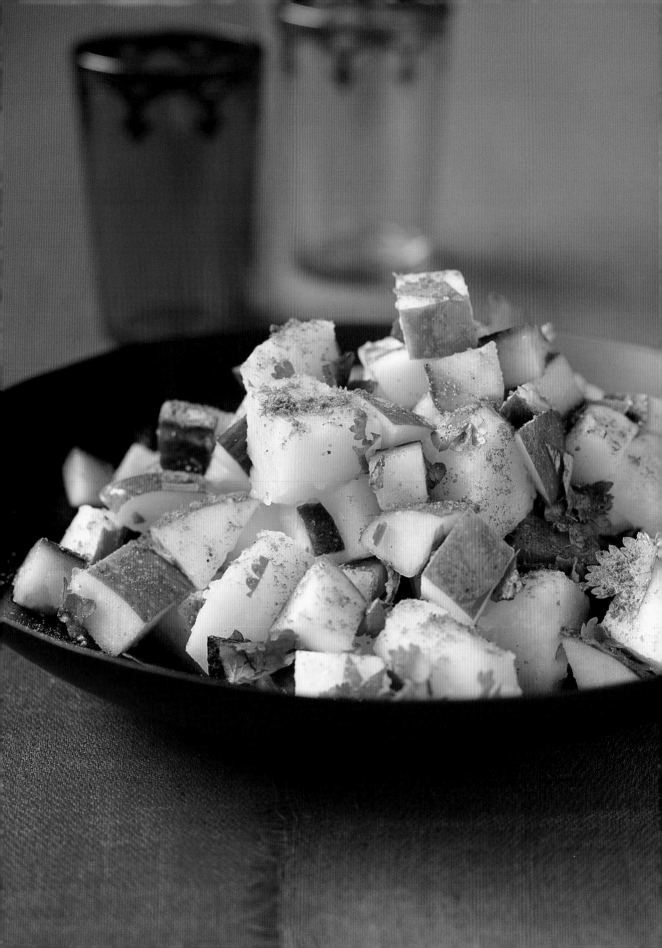

GUJARATI CARROT SALAD

This crunchy, colourful salad from Gujarat uses freshly grated carrots, lightly flavoured with mustard seeds and lime juice – a perfect foil to a spicy curry!

SERVES 4 Ⓥ
Syns per serving
Green: Free
Original: Free

EXTRA EASY
Preparation time 10 minutes
Cooking time 1 minute

600g/1lb 6oz carrots, peeled and coarsely grated

juice of 2 limes

½ tsp artificial sweetener

Fry Light

1 tbsp black mustard seeds

salt and freshly ground black pepper

1. Place the carrots in a mixing bowl. Mix together the lime juice and sweetener and stir into the grated carrot, toss to combine the ingredients well and set aside.

2. Liberally spray a small frying pan with Fry Light and place over a medium heat. Add the mustard seeds and when they start to pop (this will only take a few seconds) empty the contents of the frying pan onto the carrot mixture. Toss to combine, season and serve immediately.

FRESH TOMATO AND
MINT SALAD

In this refreshing salad of tomatoes and mint, lightly roasted cumin and mustard seeds are a welcome addition to the whole flavour of the dish.

SERVES 4 ⓥ
Syns per serving
Green: Free
Original: Free
EASY
Preparation time 10 minutes
Cooking time 1 minute

700g/1lb 8oz ripe tomatoes, thinly sliced
a handful of mint leaves
salt and freshly ground black pepper
¼ tsp mild chilli powder
juice of 1 large lemon
Fry Light
1 tsp cumin seeds
1 tsp black mustard seeds

1. Arrange the tomato slices in overlapping layers on a large plate. Tuck the mint leaves in between the tomato slices. Season well with salt, pepper and chilli powder and pour the lemon juice over.

2. Spray a frying pan with Fry Light and place over a medium heat. Add the cumin and mustard seeds and when the mustard seeds start to pop (this will only take a few seconds), lift the frying pan off the heat and spoon the spices over the tomato mixture. Serve immediately.

CUCUMBER AND CURRY LEAF SALAD

MEDIUM

Curry leaf is widely used as a flavouring in Indian cooking and is available in Asian greengrocers or in large supermarkets. Try to find fresh curry leaves and freeze any leftovers. They freeze really well and don't need defrosting before using.

SERVES 4 ⓥ
Syns per serving
Green: 1
Original: 1
EASY
Preparation time 5 minutes
Cooking time 5 minutes

1 large cucumber, peeled and finely chopped

juice of 1 lemon

salt

Fry Light

1 tsp yellow mustard seeds

½ tsp black mustard seeds

8–10 fresh curry leaves

1–2 fresh red chillies, deseeded and finely chopped

1 tbsp finely chopped roasted peanuts

1. Place the cucumber in a large mixing bowl, sprinkle over the lemon juice and season with salt. Stir to mix well and set aside.

2. Liberally spray a pan with Fry Light and place over a medium heat. Add the yellow and black mustard seeds, curry leaves and red chilli and stir-fry for 1–2 minutes. Remove from the heat and add to the cucumber mixture.

3. Toss to mix well, sprinkle over the chopped peanuts and serve immediately.

SPICED MUSHROOM AND CORIANDER SALAD

MEDIUM

This is a great way to eat mushrooms – they marry well with the aromatic spicy coriander, zesty lemon, onion and chilli.

SERVES 4 Ⓥ
Syns per serving
Green: 1½
Original: 1½
EXTRA EASY
Preparation time 10 minutes
Cooking time none

400g/14oz baby button mushrooms, halved lengthways

1 small red onion, peeled, halved and thinly sliced

a small handful of roughly chopped coriander leaves

3 tbsp lemon juice

1 tbsp sunflower oil or light olive oil

1 fresh green chilli, deseeded and finely chopped

salt

1. Place the mushrooms in a mixing bowl with the onion and coriander leaves. Set aside.

2. Mix together the remaining ingredients to make the dressing. Pour over the mushroom mixture, toss to mix well and serve immediately.

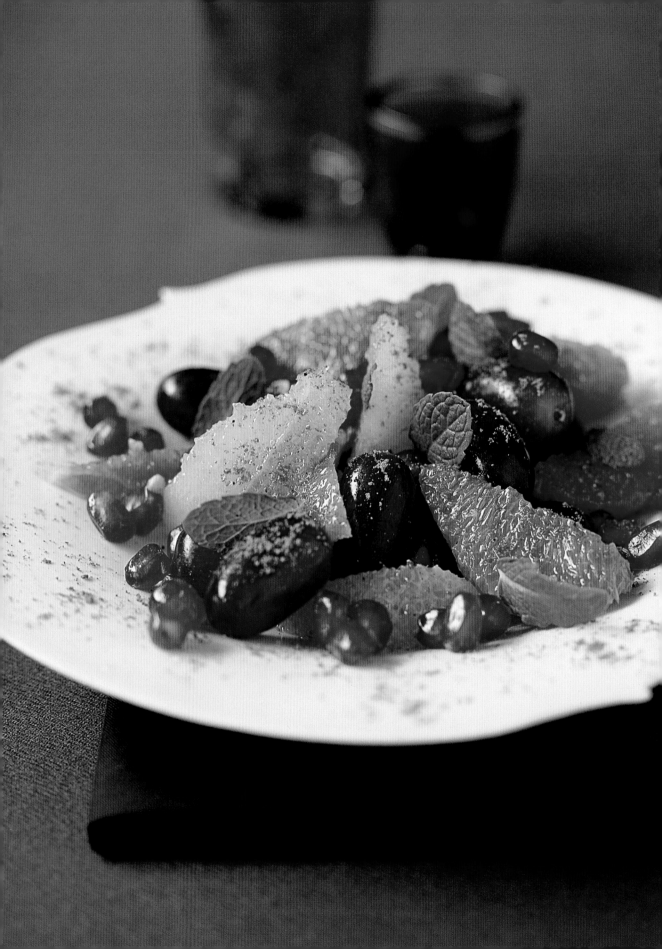

SPICED MIXED FRUIT SALAD

MILD ✦

Spiced fruit salads are often served alongside main dishes, but can be eaten on their own either at the start or end of the meal. Experiment with any variety of fruits that you like!

SERVES 4 Ⓥ
Syns per serving
Green: Free
Original: Free

EASY
Preparation time 5 minutes
(plus chilling)
Cooking time none

2 pomegranates, skin and pith removed

1 pink grapefruit, peeled and segmented

2 large oranges, peeled and segmented

200g/7oz seedless black grapes

1 tbsp chat masala

TO SERVE
a handful of mint leaves

1. Place the fruit in a serving bowl and sprinkle over the chat masala. Cover and chill in the fridge for 20–30 minutes.

2. Just before serving, add the mint leaves and toss well to combine. Serve immediately.

TIP Chat masala is a blend of spices that has a fresh taste with bitter notes. It's very versatile and tastes great in vegetable- and fruit-based dishes. If you fancy making your own, see the recipe for Aloo chat on page 70.

PAPAYA AND CHILLI RAITA

MEDIUM 〃

This nutritious and juicy tropical fruit has a sweet flavour and is packed with betacarotene. Here it is turned into a simple refreshing salad that is a good accompaniment to any spicy main dish.

SERVES 4 Ⓥ

Syns per serving
Green: Free
Original: Free

EXTRA EASY
Preparation time 5 minutes
Cooking time none

700g/1lb 8oz ripe papaya

2 fresh red chillies, deseeded and finely chopped

150g pot very low fat natural yogurt

2 tsp roasted cumin seeds, crushed

salt

a pinch of mild or medium chilli powder

1. Cut the papaya in half lengthways and scoop out the seeds. Peel off the skin with a sharp knife and cut the flesh into 1.5cm/½in cubes. Place in a mixing bowl with the red chilli.

2. Place the yogurt in a bowl and stir in the crushed cumin seeds. Season well with salt, then pour this mixture over the papaya and stir to coat evenly. Sprinkle over the chilli powder and serve.

SWEETCORN RAITA

Raitas are salads with a yogurt dressing and are usually lightly spiced. Fresh or canned sweetcorn kernels can be used in this wonderfully different salad, which is a great accompaniment to any meal.

SERVES 4 Ⓥ
Syns per serving
Green: Free

EASY
Preparation time 10 minutes
Cooking time 10 minutes

Fry Light

1 tsp black mustard seeds

1 tsp peeled and finely chopped garlic

1 tsp peeled and finely chopped ginger

1 fresh red chilli, deseeded and finely chopped

½ red pepper, deseeded and finely chopped

400g/14oz fresh or canned sweetcorn kernels

salt

250g pot very low fat natural yogurt

2 tbsp finely chopped coriander leaves

1. Spray a large, non-stick frying pan with Fry Light and place over a moderate heat. Add the mustard seeds, garlic, ginger and red chilli and stir-fry for 2–3 minutes.

2. Stir in the chopped red pepper and sweetcorn with 2–3 table-spoons of water and continue to stir-fry for 3–4 minutes. Season with salt, remove from the heat and allow to cool.

3. Beat the yogurt until smooth and place in a large bowl. Add the sweetcorn mixture and the chopped coriander and stir to mix well. Serve immediately.

LEMONGRASS PRAWN SALAD MEDIUM

This refreshing salad is of Thai origin but the addition of curry powder gives it an Indo-Thai twist.

SERVES 4
Syns per serving
Green: 3
Original: Free

EASY
Preparation time 10 minutes
Cooking time 10 minutes

4 tbsp chicken stock made with Bovril

2 tbsp nam pla

2 tsp mild or medium curry powder

24 tiger prawns

1 tbsp very finely chopped lemongrass

3 small shallots, peeled and very finely chopped

¼ tsp artificial sweetener

2 tbsp lemon juice

2 spring onions, trimmed and finely chopped

1 small cucumber, cut into thin shreds with a vegetable peeler

1 carrot, peeled and cut into thin shreds with a vegetable peeler

TO SERVE
light soy sauce

1. Place the stock, nam pla and curry powder in a saucepan and bring to the boil. Add the prawns and cook for 3–4 minutes or until opaque and just cooked through.

2. Add the remaining ingredients, stir and cook for 1 minute and then remove from the heat.

3. Divide the warmed salad between four warmed bowls and serve immediately with light soy sauce to drizzle over.

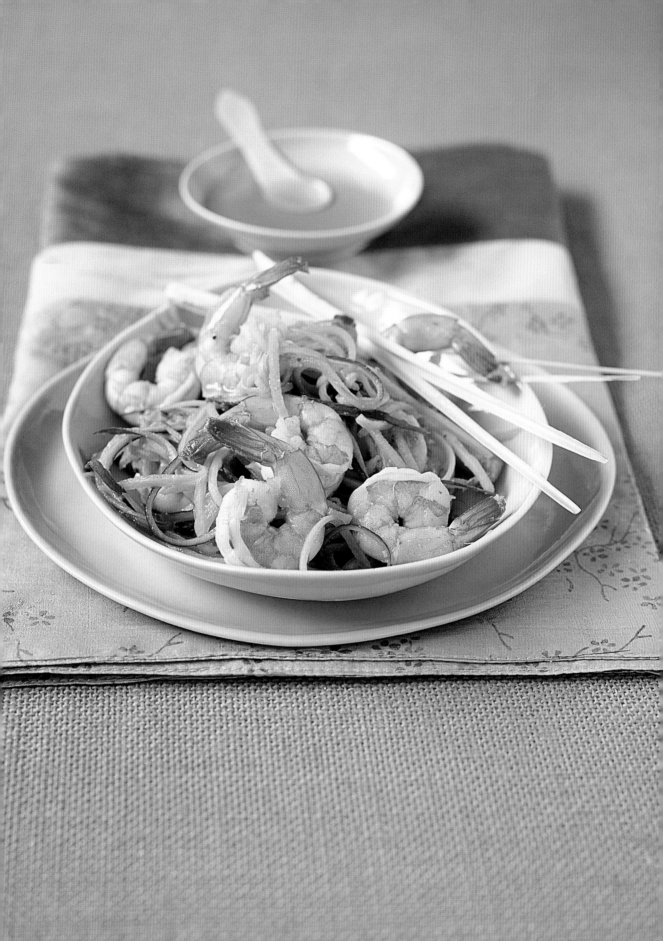

SPICED MIXED SPROUTED BEAN SALAD

MEDIUM 🌶🌶

Packets of mixed sprouted beans are now widely available in supermarkets and good greengrocers. They comprise a mixture of sprouted mung beans, chickpeas, aduki beans and lentil sprouts. Known in India as 'living food', sprouted beans are extremely healthy and nutritious and this salad is a classic favourite.

SERVES 4 Ⓥ
Syns per serving
Green: Free
EASY
Preparation time 5 minutes
Cooking time 5 minutes

Fry Light
1 tsp black mustard seeds
1 tsp cumin seeds
1 tsp peeled and finely grated ginger
1 fresh red chilli, deseeded and finely chopped or sliced
400g/14oz mixed sprouted beans
1 tsp mild or medium chilli powder
juice of 1 lime
salt
3 tbsp very low fat natural yogurt

TO SERVE
chicory leaves

1. Spray a large frying pan with Fry Light and place over a medium heat. Add the mustard and cumin seeds and when the mustard seeds start to pop (this won't take long), stir in the ginger, red chilli and sprouted beans.

2. Stir-fry for 2–3 minutes, then add the chilli powder. Remove from the heat and squeeze over the lime juice. Season well with salt and allow to cool.

3. When cool, stir in the yogurt, mix well and serve immediately on a bed of chicory leaves.

CHICKEN TIKKA AND RED ONION SALAD

Tikka means marinated and then grilled or baked. Here chicken tikka pieces are served in a delicious salad with red onions and mixed baby salad leaves.

SERVES 4
Syns per serving
Original: Free
EASY
Preparation time 10 minutes
(plus marinating)
Cooking time 20 minutes

1 tsp peeled and finely grated ginger

3 garlic cloves, peeled and crushed

1 tsp hot chilli powder

¼ tsp turmeric

150g pot very low fat natural yogurt

juice of 1 lemon

1 tbsp finely chopped coriander leaves

salt

4 chicken breasts, skinless and boneless, cut into bite-sized chunks

Fry Light

TO SERVE

1 red onion, peeled and thinly sliced

110g/4oz mixed baby salad leaves

lemon wedges

1. Mix together the ginger, garlic, chilli powder, turmeric, yogurt, lemon juice and coriander leaves. Season well with salt and pour the marinade over the chicken. Toss to mix well, cover and leave to marinate in the fridge overnight.

2. Place the chicken on a grill rack and spray with Fry Light. Cook under a medium-hot grill for 15–20 minutes, turning occasionally, until cooked through. Remove and allow to cool.

3. Toss the onion and baby salad leaves together and divide between four salad plates. Top each salad with the cooked chicken and serve immediately with lemon wedges.

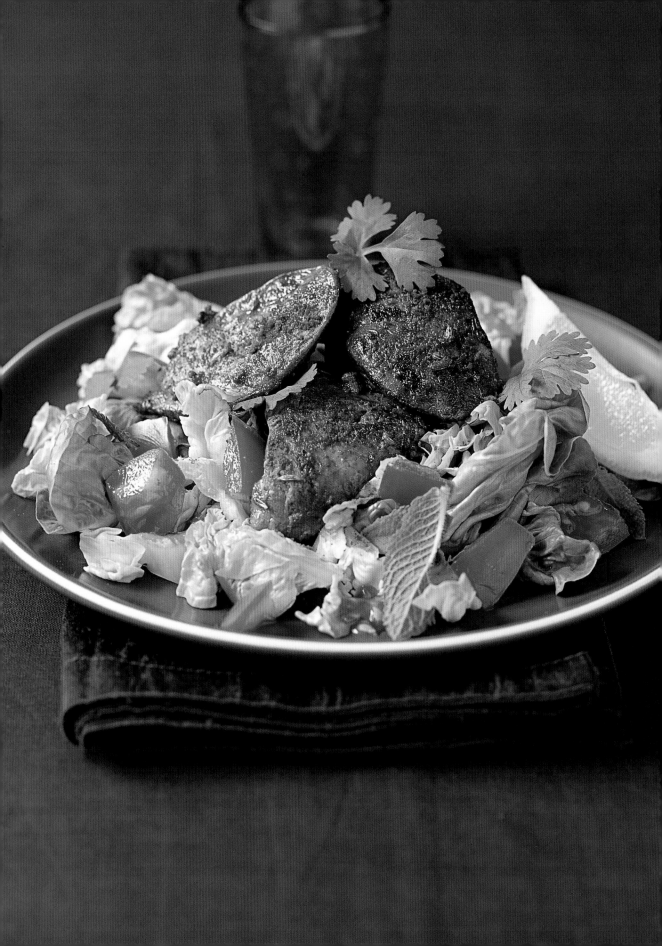

WARMED CURRIED CHICKEN LIVER SALAD

Chicken livers are a delicacy and widely eaten in India simply seared. Here, coupled with fresh coriander and mint, they make a wonderful warm salad.

SERVES 4
Syns per serving
Original: Free

EASY
Preparation time 10 minutes
Cooking time 5 minutes

a large handful of coriander leaves

a large handful of mint leaves

2 baby gem lettuces, leaves separated and shredded

4 midi plum tomatoes, roughly chopped

450g/1lb chicken livers, trimmed

1 tsp ground cumin

1 tsp ground coriander

½ tsp mild or medium chilli powder

1 tsp crushed fennel seeds

1 tsp peeled and crushed garlic

1 tsp peeled and finely grated ginger

2 tbsp white vinegar

salt and freshly ground black pepper

Fry Light

a pinch of paprika

TO SERVE
lemon wedges

1. Mix together the coriander, mint, lettuce leaves and tomatoes and set aside.

2. Place the chicken livers in a bowl. Mix the cumin, coriander, chilli, fennel, garlic and ginger with the vinegar to make a smooth paste. Season well and then spread the mixture over the livers to coat completely.

3. Spray a pan with Fry Light and place over a high heat. Add the chicken livers and stir-fry for 3–4 minutes or until the livers are lightly browned. (Take care not to overcook them as they should be slightly pink on the inside.)

4. Divide the coriander, mint and lettuce mixture between four plates, top with the curried chicken livers and sprinkle over the paprika. Serve warm with lemon wedges to squeeze over.

CITRUS PORK SALAD

MEDIUM ✌

Minced pork is quickly cooked with spices and then served with chunks of orange and lettuce leaves in this refreshing salad that teases the taste buds. If liked, minced beef or chicken could be used as an alternative to the pork.

SERVES 4
Syns per serving
Original: ½

EASY
Preparation time 10 minutes
Cooking time 10 minutes

Fry Light

1 small onion, peeled and finely chopped

2 garlic cloves, peeled and finely chopped

1 tsp peeled and finely grated ginger

2 tsp medium curry powder

250g/9oz lean minced pork

salt and freshly ground black pepper

juice of 1 orange

TO SERVE

2 large oranges, peeled and segmented

2 baby gem lettuces, leaves separated

red pepper strips

1. Spray a large pan with Fry Light and place over a medium heat. Add the onion, garlic and ginger and stir-fry for 3–4 minutes.

2. Add the curry powder and pork and stir-fry over a high heat for 5–6 minutes or until the pork is browned and cooked through. Remove from the heat and season well. Stir in the orange juice and allow to cool.

3. Meanwhile, divide the orange segments and lettuce leaves between four serving plates. Top with the pork mixture, garnish with red pepper strips and serve immediately.

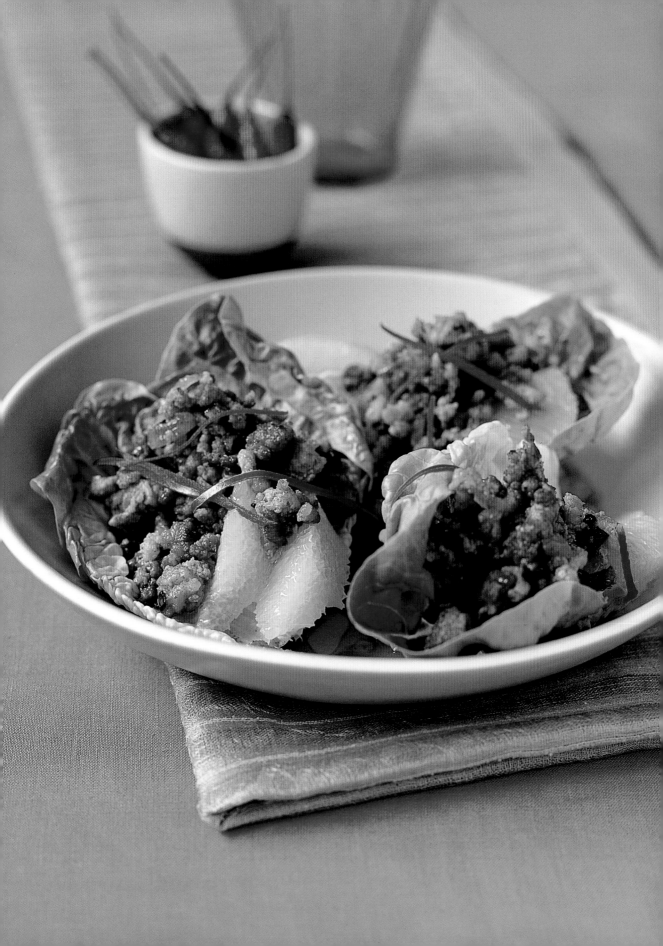

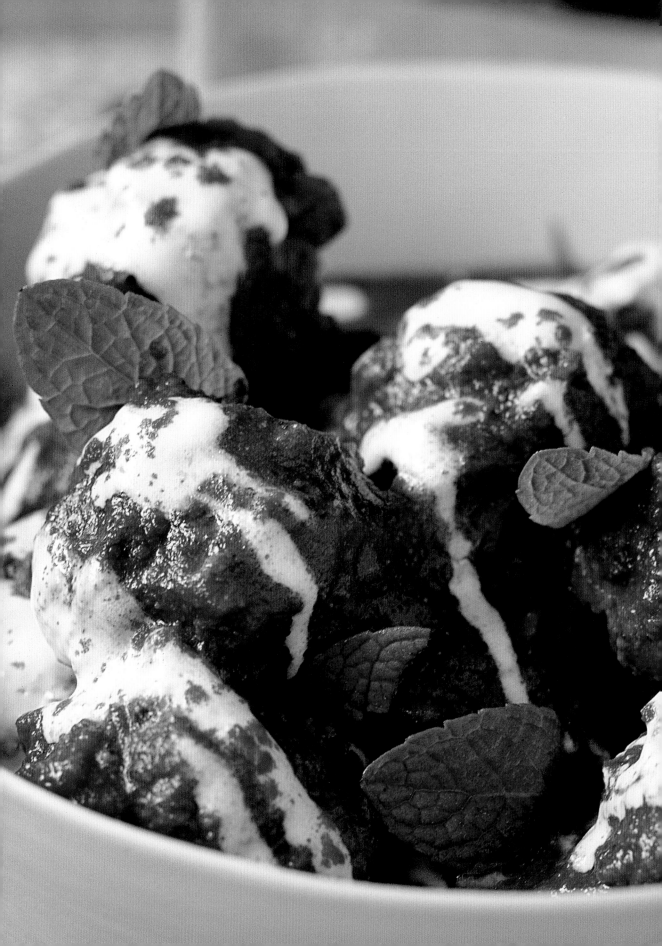

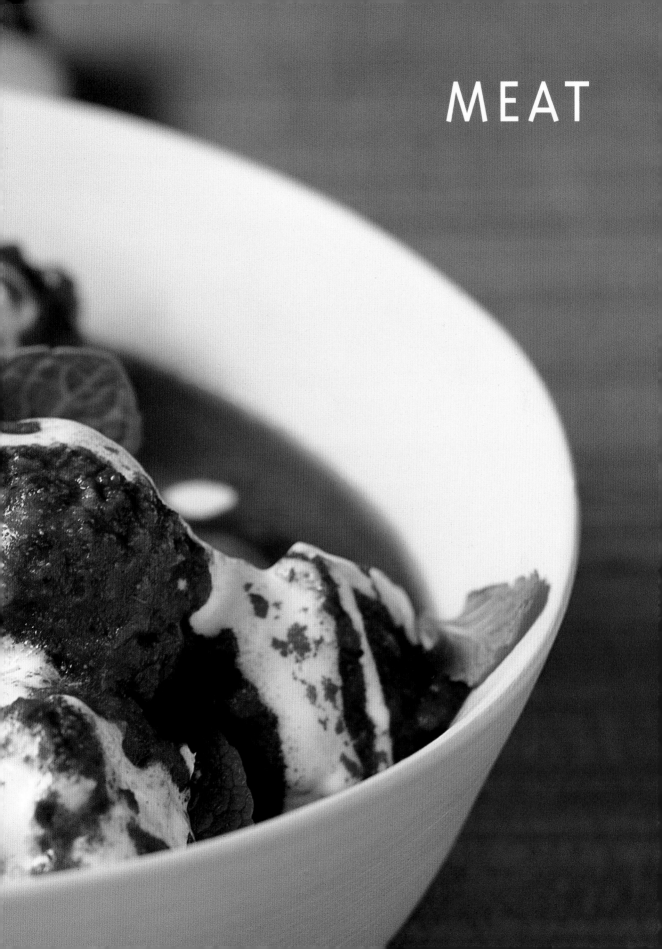

MEAT

KHEEMA WITH CURRY LEAVES

MEDIUM

In this quick and easy to prepare Indian-style stir-fry, lean pork mince is cooked in its own juices and delicately flavoured with fresh curry leaves.

SERVES 4
Syns per serving
Original: Free

EXTRA EASY
Preparation time 15 minutes
Cooking time 20 minutes

Fry Light

1 large onion, peeled and finely chopped

10–12 fresh curry leaves

2 fresh green chillies, deseeded and chopped

400g/14oz lean minced pork

3 garlic cloves, peeled and crushed

1 tsp peeled and finely grated ginger

1 tsp mild chilli powder

¼ tsp turmeric

1 tsp salt

3–4 ripe tomatoes, quartered

4 tbsp freshly chopped coriander leaves

1. Spray a frying pan with Fry Light and place over a medium heat. Add the onion, curry leaves and chillies and stir-fry for 2–3 minutes.

2. Place the minced pork in a bowl along with the garlic, ginger, chilli powder, turmeric and salt. Mix thoroughly using your fingers. Add this mixture to the frying pan and stir-fry over a high heat for 7–10 minutes.

3. Add the tomatoes and coriander and continue to fry for 3–4 minutes. Remove from the heat and serve with Garam masala tamatar (see page 187).

TIP If you can't find curry leaves, use 1–2 fresh bay leaves instead. This dish would make a great talking point at a dinner party if you served it on a banana leaf – only you need know how easy it is to create!

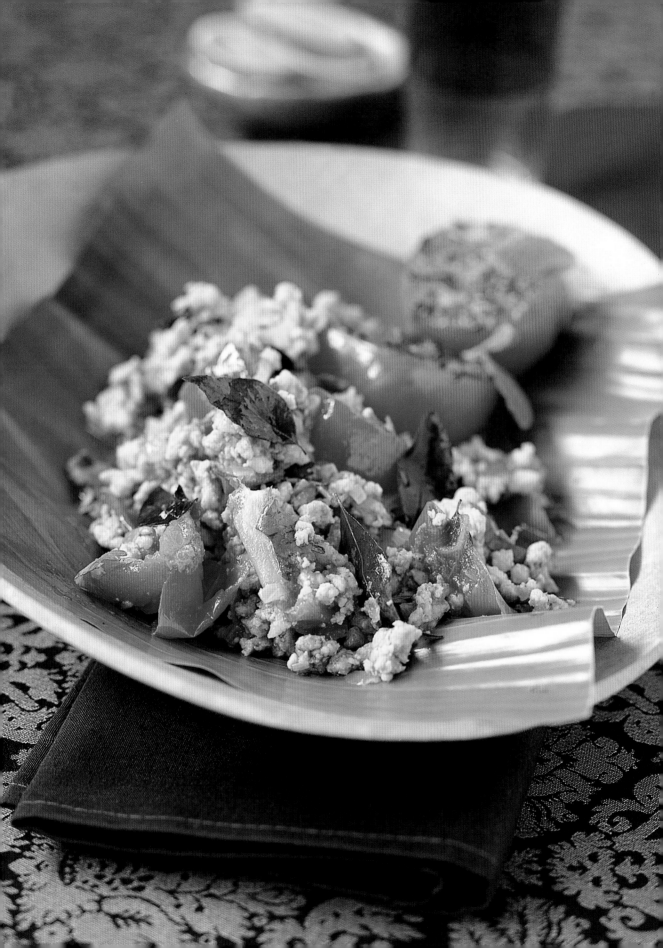

SPICY PORK AND PARSNIP STEW

MEDIUM 🌶🌶

This hearty, spicy stew is perfect for a warming supper. You could use lamb as a substitute for the pork if preferred.

SERVES 4 ❄
Syns per serving
Original: 1½
EASY
Preparation time 20 minutes
Cooking time 1 hour 50 minutes

Fry Light

1 onion, peeled and finely chopped

2 bay leaves

1 fresh red chilli, deseeded and finely chopped

2 garlic cloves, peeled and finely chopped

700g/1lb 8oz pork fillet, all visible fat removed, cut into bite-sized chunks

2 tsp ground coriander

1 tsp ground cumin

½ tsp turmeric

½ tsp mild or medium chilli powder

½ tsp ground cinnamon

salt and freshly ground black pepper

250g/9oz tomatoes, finely chopped

700ml/24fl oz chicken stock made with Bovril

175g/6oz parsnips, peeled and cut into bite-sized chunks

1. Spray a saucepan with Fry Light and place over a medium heat. Add the onion, bay leaves, red chilli and garlic and stir-fry for 4–5 minutes.

2. Turn the heat to high and add the pork to the saucepan. Cook, stirring continuously, for 6–8 minutes or until lightly browned. Add the coriander, cumin, turmeric, chilli powder and cinnamon, season well and cook, continuing to stir, for 3–4 minutes.

3. Add the tomatoes and stock, bring to the boil, cover, reduce the heat to low and simmer gently for 1 hour, stirring occasionally.

4. Add the parsnips and cook for a further 25–30 minutes or until the meat and parsnips are tender. Remove from the heat and serve ladled into warmed bowls.

TIP Make this dish Free on Original days by swapping the parsnips for celeriac.

ADRAKHWALA CHOPS

MEDIUM 🌶️🌶️

These lean pork chops, marinated with ginger, vinegar and chilli, are cooked slowly in the oven until deliciously tender.

SERVES 4 ❄️
Syns per serving
Original: Free
EASY
Preparation time 15 minutes
(plus marinating)
Cooking time 1 hour

1 tbsp peeled and finely grated ginger

1 tbsp peeled and finely grated garlic

2 tbsp vinegar

2 tsp mild or medium chilli powder

¼ tsp artificial sweetener

8 pork chops, all visible fat removed

salt

1. Place the ginger, garlic, vinegar, chilli powder and sweetener in a small bowl and mix together.

2. Place the pork chops in a single layer in an ovenproof casserole dish. Spread the ginger mixture evenly over the chops, season with salt, cover and leave to marinate in the fridge overnight.

3. Preheat the oven 180°C/Gas 4. Pour 200ml/7fl oz of water around the pork, cover tightly, place in the oven and cook for 1 hour or until cooked through and tender. Remove from the oven and serve with the pan juices spooned over.

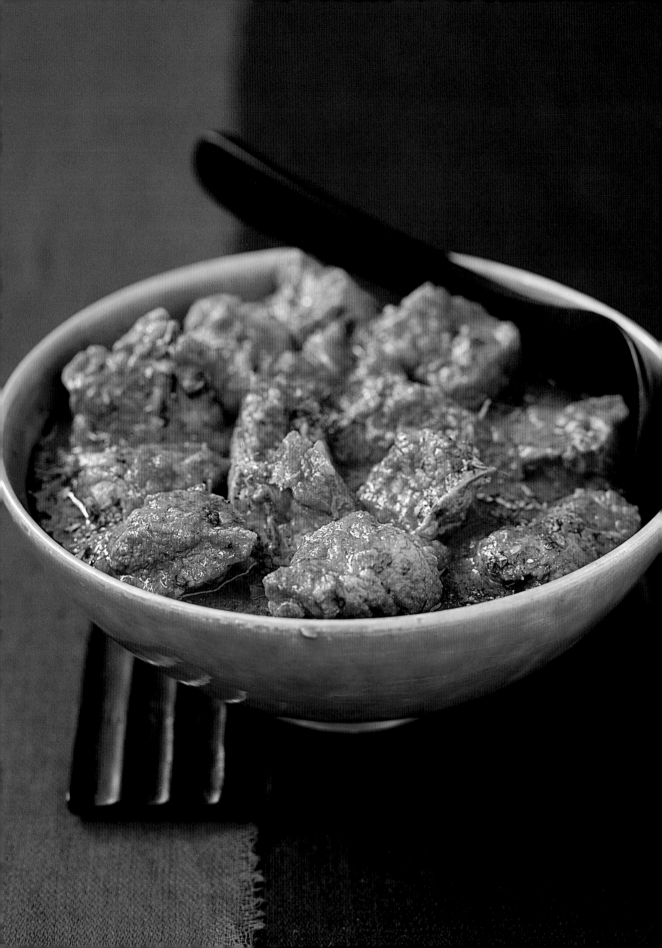

PORK VINDALOO

This dish comes from the coastal state of Goa and is a speciality of the area. Vindaloo dishes always have vinegar as one of the main ingredients.

SERVES 4 ❅
Syns per serving
Original: Free

EASY
Preparation time 15 minutes
(plus marinating)
Cooking time 1 hour 15 minutes

500g/1lb 2oz pork, all visible fat removed, cut into bite-sized chunks

125ml/4fl oz vinegar

1 onion, peeled and grated

2 tsp ground cumin

2 tsp ground black mustard seeds

8 garlic cloves, peeled and crushed

2 tsp peeled and finely grated ginger

2 tsp hot chilli powder

½ tsp ground cloves

1 tsp ground cinnamon

Fry Light

400g can chopped tomatoes

¼ tsp artificial sweetener

salt and freshly ground black pepper

TO SERVE
freshly chopped coriander leaves

1. Place the pork in a bowl. Mix 1 tablespoon vinegar with a little water and pour over. Toss to coat.

2. Place the remaining vinegar in a bowl with the onion, cumin, mustard seeds, garlic, ginger, chilli, cloves and cinnamon. Mix well to form a smooth paste and pour over the pork to coat evenly. Cover the bowl and leave to marinate in the fridge for 6–8 hours or overnight if time permits.

3. Spray a saucepan with Fry Light and place over a high heat. To the pan, add 200ml/7fl oz of water, the pork mixture, tomatoes and sweetener and bring to the boil. Reduce the heat to low, season well, cover tightly and simmer gently for about an hour or until the pork is tender.

4. Remove from the heat and allow to rest for 10 minutes before serving with freshly chopped coriander scattered over.

SHISH PATTIES

Minced lamb is marinated with yogurt and spices and quickly grilled to perfection. You could use any other type of lean mince if you prefer.

SERVES 4 ❄
Syns per serving
Original: Free
EXTRA EASY
Preparation time 15 minutes
(plus marinating)
Cooking time 15 minutes

4 garlic cloves, peeled and crushed

1 tsp peeled and finely grated ginger

1 tsp hot chilli powder

1 red chilli, finely chopped

1 tsp ground coriander

2 tsp ground cumin

1 tsp ground cinnamon

¼ tsp ground cloves

¼ tsp ground cardamom

2 tbsp finely chopped shallots

500g/1lb 2oz extra-lean minced lamb

2 tbsp very low fat natural yogurt

salt and freshly ground black pepper

Fry Light

TO SERVE
lemon wedges

1. Place the garlic, ginger, chilli powder, red chilli, coriander, cumin, cinnamon, cloves, cardamom, shallots, minced lamb and yogurt in a mixing bowl. Season well and, using your fingers, combine thoroughly until well mixed. Cover and chill in the fridge for 5–6 hours (or overnight if possible) to allow the flavours to develop.

2. Divide the lamb mixture into 12 portions and form each portion into a ball. Pat each ball into a flat 'patty', place on a grill rack and lightly spray with Fry Light. Cook under a medium-hot grill for 5–6 minutes on each side or until cooked through.

3. Serve warm with wedges of lemon and a mixed salad.

TIP If you want to cheat the spices, use 1 tbsp Madras curry powder instead.

TANDOORI LAMB KEBABS

Tandoori Spice blend is a commercially sold product available in large supermarkets and Asian greengrocers and comprises a mixture of ground spices. Here the lamb is marinated in a spice paste and then grilled or barbecued until tender. Use good quality lamb (neck fillet) as it is very lean and makes for a tender and succulent kebab.

SERVES 4 ❉
Syns per serving
Original: Free

EXTRA EASY
Preparation time 15 minutes (plus marinating)
Cooking time 15 minutes

700g/1lb 8oz neck fillet of lamb, all visible fat removed

2 tsp peeled and finely grated ginger

4 garlic cloves, peeled and crushed

2 tbsp Tandoori Spice blend

200g/7oz very low fat natural yogurt

salt

2 red peppers, halved and deseeded

1. Cut the lamb into bite-sized pieces and place in a mixing bowl.

2. Mix together the ginger, garlic, Tandoori Spice blend and yogurt. Season with salt and pour over the lamb. Toss the lamb to coat completely, cover and leave to marinate in the fridge for 5–6 hours or overnight if time permits.

3. Cut the peppers into bite-sized pieces. Remove the lamb from the marinade and thread onto 12 metal skewers, alternating with the red pepper pieces. Grill under a medium-hot grill for 6–8 minutes on each side or until cooked through. Serve immediately with Brinjal Bharta (see page 206).

TIP Tandoori Spice blend is available from large supermarkets or Asian greengrocers. If you have difficulty finding it, substitute it with a hot curry powder.

LAMB ROGAN JOSH

In this mild curry, flavoured with dry-roasted spices, the lamb releases its delicious juices during a slow, gentle cooking process.

SERVES 4 ✱
Syns per serving
Original: ½

WORTH THE EFFORT
Preparation time 20 minutes
Cooking time 1 hour 20 minutes

75g/3oz very low fat natural yogurt

2 tsp mild chilli powder

2 tsp ground coriander

2 tsp ground cumin

4 garlic cloves, peeled and crushed

2 tsp peeled and finely grated ginger

½ tsp turmeric

600g/1lb 6oz lamb neck fillet or leg steak, all visible fat removed

300g/11oz onions, peeled and finely chopped

2 tbsp tomato purée

salt

Fry Light

3 dried bay leaves, crumbled

6 green cardamom pods, lightly crushed

5cm/2in cinnamon stick

4 cloves

½ tsp grated nutmeg

2 tbsp freshly chopped mint leaves

4 tbsp freshly chopped coriander leaves

1. Place the yogurt, chilli, ground coriander, cumin, garlic, ginger and turmeric in a small bowl and mix.

2. Cut the lamb into 5cm/2in cubes, place them in a large non-stick frying pan with the onions, place over a medium heat and stir until the mixture begins to sizzle. Add the yogurt mixture, reduce the heat to low, cover tightly and cook for 30 minutes, stirring occasionally, until the lamb releases its juices.

3. Uncover the pan, increase the heat to medium and cook for 5–6 minutes, stirring frequently, until the sauce has reduced to a paste-like consistency. Add the tomato purée and 350ml/12fl oz of boiling water, season with salt, cover and leave to simmer for 15–20 minutes.

4. Spray a small frying pan with Fry Light and place over a low heat. Add the bay leaves, cardamom, cinnamon and cloves and allow to sizzle for 40–45 seconds. Pour the contents of this pan over the meat along with the nutmeg, stir to mix, cover tightly and cook gently for another 12–15 minutes or until the meat is tender. Remove from the heat and stir in the fresh mint and coriander before serving.

TIP Don't let the amount of spices used in this dish put you off – you could use 1 tbsp medium curry powder instead if you want.

SHISH KEBABS

Lean minced lamb is blended to a paste with yogurt, spices and fresh coriander, then moulded around skewers to make tasty kebabs. For a special occasion, use lemongrass stalks – the kebabs will look sensational.

SERVES 4 ❄

Syns per serving
Original: 2

EASY
Preparation time 10 minutes
Cooking time 10 minutes

1.5cm/½in cube ginger, peeled and chopped

1 garlic clove, peeled and chopped

500g/1lb 2oz lean minced lamb

a small bunch coriander leaves, stalks removed and chopped

1 tbsp amchoor (dried mango powder), or lemon juice

1 tsp garam masala

1 tsp ground cumin

1 tsp mild or medium chilli powder

2 tbsp gram flour

2 tbsp very low fat natural yogurt

salt and freshly ground black pepper

Fry Light

TO SERVE
lemon wedges
freshly chopped coriander leaves

1. Put the ginger and garlic in a food processor with the lamb. Add the chopped coriander, amchoor or lemon juice, spices, flour and yogurt and blend to a paste. Transfer to a bowl and season well with salt and pepper.

2. Preheat the grill. Divide the mixture into 8 portions and mould each into a sausage around a metal skewer. Spray with Fry Light and grill for 8–10 minutes, turning once. Serve immediately with lemon wedges and sprinkled with chopped coriander.

DAHIWALLA GHOSHT

MILD

Trimmed racks of lamb are available in large supermarkets, but if you're unable to find them, your local butcher will happily 'French trim' the lamb for you. The spiced yogurt mixture tenderises the meat as it marinates, so it's a good idea to marinate the lamb for as long as possible to give you a moist, succulent flavour and texture.

SERVES 4
Syns per serving
Original: Free
EASY
Preparation time 10 minutes
(plus marinating)
Cooking time 25 minutes

4 trimmed racks of lamb

3 garlic cloves, peeled and crushed

2 tsp peeled and finely grated ginger

2 tbsp white wine vinegar

2 tbsp dried mint

3 tsp ground cumin

2 tsp ground coriander

1 tsp mild chilli powder

150g pot very low fat natural yogurt

salt and freshly ground black pepper

1. Place the racks of lamb in a single layer in a shallow bowl. Place all the remaining ingredients in a food processor, season well and blend until smooth. Pour this mixture over the lamb to coat evenly. Cover and leave to marinate overnight in the fridge to allow the flavours to develop.

2. Remove the lamb from the fridge 1 hour before cooking. Preheat the oven to 200°C/Gas 6, place the lamb on a non-stick baking sheet and bake for 20–25 minutes or until cooked to your liking.

3. Remove the lamb from the oven, cover with foil and allow to rest for 5–10 minutes before carving each rack into cutlets. Serve immediately with Kachumber (see page 212).

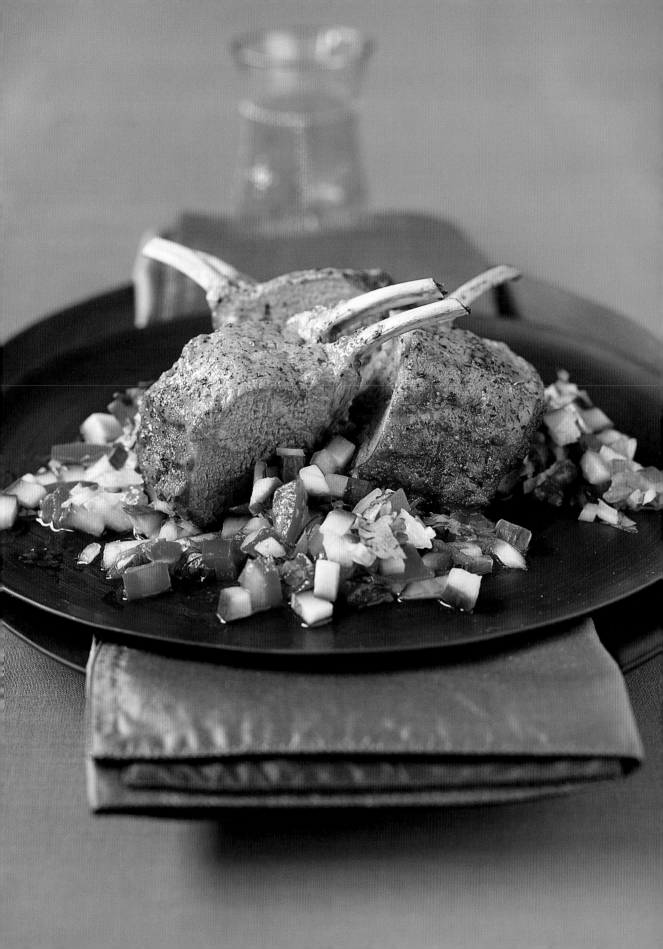

CINNAMON AND CORIANDER LAMB SHANKS

MILD ✒

This wonderful entertaining dish of lamb shanks is delicately flavoured with spices and slowly cooked until the meat is meltingly tender. Trim all visible fat from the shanks, or get your butcher to do this for you. You need a heavy-based, large casserole dish with a tight-fitting lid for this recipe.

SERVES 4 ❄

Syns per serving
Original: Free

EXTRA EASY
Preparation time 10 minutes
Cooking time 2 hours 45 minutes

4 lamb shanks, all visible fat removed

1 onion, peeled and roughly chopped

8 garlic cloves, peeled

2 tsp peeled and finely grated ginger

5–6 fresh curry leaves

1 tbsp ground coriander

2 tsp ground cinnamon

400g can chopped tomatoes

1 tsp mild chilli powder

¼ tsp artificial sweetener

600ml/1 pint chicken stock made with Bovril

salt

TO SERVE
freshly chopped coriander leaves

1. Place the lamb shanks in a deep, heavy-based casserole dish to fit snugly. Mix all the remaining ingredients together and add to the dish.

2. Bring the mixture to the boil, cover tightly, reduce the heat to very low and simmer for 2 hours, checking from time to time that the mixture is simmering gently.

3. Uncover the dish and continue to simmer for 30–45 minutes until the meat is almost coming off the bone.

4. Remove the dish from the heat and allow to stand for 5–10 minutes before serving garnished with freshly chopped coriander leaves.

RAAN OF LAMB

This northern Indian-frontier speciality comprises a leg of lamb that has been marinated for 24 hours in a delicate spice mixture and then slowly roasted in the oven.

SERVES 4
Syns per serving
Original: Free
EASY
Preparation time 20 minutes
(plus marinating)
Cooking time 2 hours 15 minutes

1.5kg/3lb 6oz leg of lamb, all visible fat removed

2 tsp mild or medium chilli powder

2 garlic cloves, peeled and crushed

3 tsp ground coriander

2 tsp ground cumin

1 tsp ground cloves

2 tsp ground cinnamon

10 tbsp very low fat natural yogurt

salt and freshly ground black pepper

1. Place the lamb in a large dish and, using a sharp knife, make deep cuts all over the flesh (to allow the marinade to penetrate deeply).

2. Mix all the remaining ingredients together to make the marinade. Pour over the lamb and rub into the flesh. Cover and chill for 24 hours to allow the flavours to develop and the meat to tenderise.

3. Remove the lamb from the fridge 1 hour before cooking to allow it to reach room temperature. Preheat the oven to 180°C/Gas 4. Place the lamb in a non-stick roasting tray and spoon any remaining marinade over. Cover loosely with foil and bake for 1½ hours.

4. Remove the foil and baste the lamb with the pan juices. Return to the oven uncovered for another 40–45 minutes or until cooked to your liking. Remove from the oven, cover with foil and allow to rest for 10–15 minutes before carving into thin slices and serving.

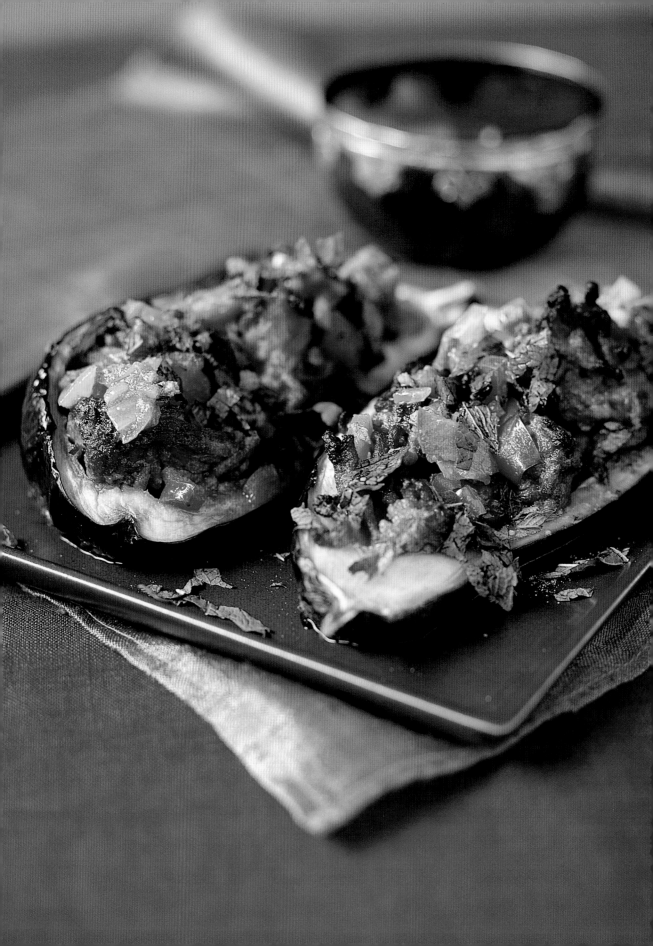

STUFFED AUBERGINES WITH SPICED LAMB

HOT 🌶🌶🌶

Aubergines and spiced minced lamb are a combination that marries very well. Here, spiced minced lamb is stuffed into halved aubergine shells and baked to perfection.

SERVES 4 ❄
Syns per serving
Original: Free
EASY
Preparation time 20 minutes
Cooking time 45 minutes

2 aubergines

Fry Light

1 onion, peeled and thinly sliced

1 tsp peeled and finely grated ginger

1 tsp hot chilli powder

2 garlic cloves, peeled and crushed

¼ tsp turmeric

2 tsp salt

1 tsp ground coriander

2 tsp dried mint

1 ripe tomato, finely chopped

450g/1lb extra-lean minced lamb

1 red pepper, deseeded and finely diced

2 tbsp freshly chopped coriander leaves

2 tbsp freshly chopped mint leaves

TO SERVE
ground cumin

1. Preheat the oven to 180°C/Gas 4. Cut the aubergines in half lengthways and, using a sharp knife and a spoon, scoop out most of the flesh and discard. Place the aubergine shells, cut side up, on a baking sheet and set aside until needed.

2. Spray a large frying pan with Fry Light and place over a medium heat. Add the onions and stir-fry for 4–5 minutes. Then add the ginger, chilli powder, garlic, turmeric, salt, ground coriander, dried mint and chopped tomato and stir-fry for 4–5 minutes.

3. Add the minced lamb and continue to stir-fry for 5–6 minutes over a high heat. Add the diced pepper, freshly chopped coriander and mint, stir to mix well and remove from the heat.

4. Carefully spoon the lamb mixture into the prepared aubergine shells. Lightly spray each one with Fry Light and bake for 20–25 minutes. Remove from the oven and serve immediately, sprinkled with ground cumin.

ELAICHI GHOSHT

This mild and aromatic lamb dish comes from the Sindhi community of northern India. Elaichi is the Indian name for cardamom. Serve with a selection of steamed Free vegetables for a veritable feast.

SERVES 4 ❄

Syns per serving
Original: ½

EASY

Preparation time 15 minutes
Cooking time 1 hour 30 minutes

900g/2lb lamb, all visible fat removed, cut into bite-sized chunks

1 tbsp ground cardamom seeds

2 large tomatoes, roughly chopped

2 red onions, peeled and finely chopped

2 tsp garam masala

2 tbsp tomato purée

salt and freshly ground black pepper

1. Place the lamb in a bowl, sprinkle over the cardamom seeds and toss to mix well. Transfer to a heavy-based saucepan along with the tomatoes, onion, garam masala and tomato purée.

2. Pour over 700ml/24fl oz of water, season well and bring the mixture to the boil. Cover tightly, reduce the heat to low and cook for 1½ hours, stirring occasionally until the meat is tender.

3. Remove the saucepan from the heat and allow to stand for 5 minutes before serving.

MAGALOREAN TOMATO AND BEEF CURRY

HOT 〟〟〟

Though the list of ingredients in this recipe may be long, do not be intimidated by it as it is really easy to make, the preparation time is quite painless and the result is scrumptious.

SERVES 4 ❋
Syns per serving
Original: 1

EXTRA EASY
Preparation time 15 minutes
Cooking time 1 hour 40 minutes

500g/1lb 2oz beef, all visible fat removed, cut into bite-sized chunks

1 onion, peeled and finely chopped

1 tsp peeled and finely grated ginger

4 garlic cloves, peeled and crushed

400g can chopped tomatoes

a large handful of freshly chopped coriander leaves

2 fresh red chillies, sliced

¼ tsp turmeric

2 tsp garam masala

2 tsp ground cumin

4 tbsp reduced-fat coconut milk

1 tbsp tomato purée

salt and freshly ground black pepper

TO SERVE
110g/4oz very low fat natural yogurt

1. Place all the ingredients in a non-stick saucepan together with 350ml/12fl oz of water. Place over a high heat and bring to the boil. Cover tightly, reduce the heat to low and simmer gently for 1½ hours or until the meat is tender.

2. Uncover the pan, stir and cook over a high heat for 5–6 minutes.

3. Remove the saucepan from the heat and serve lightly drizzled with the yogurt.

TIP If you like your food hot, leave the seeds in the chillies!

BEEF KOFTA CURRY

Kofta *means meatballs in the Indian language and in this recipe beef meatballs are cooked in a smooth, spicy sauce to make a warming supper. You can use any form of lean mince that you prefer as a substitute to the beef.*

SERVES 4 ✽
Syns per serving
Original: Free
EASY
Preparation time 15 minutes
Cooking time 25 minutes

700g/1lb 8oz extra-lean minced beef
2 tsp peeled and finely grated ginger
2 garlic cloves, peeled and crushed
2 tsp crushed fennel seeds
1 tsp ground cinnamon
1 tsp mild or medium chilli powder
salt and freshly ground black pepper
1 tsp turmeric
2 tbsp medium curry powder
500ml carton passata
¼ tsp artificial sweetener

TO SERVE
very low fat natural yogurt
chilli powder
mint leaves

1. Place the minced beef in a mixing bowl along with the ginger, garlic, fennel, cinnamon and chilli powder. Season and, using your hands, mix thoroughly until well combined. Form the mixture into small, walnut-sized balls and set aside.

2. Place the turmeric, curry powder, passata and sweetener in a medium saucepan and bring to the boil. Reduce the heat to a simmer, season well and carefully place the meatballs in the sauce. Cover and cook gently for 15–20 minutes, turning the meatballs occasionally, until they are cooked through.

3. Remove from the heat and serve drizzled with very low fat natural yogurt, sprinkled with a pinch of chilli powder and garnished with fresh mint leaves.

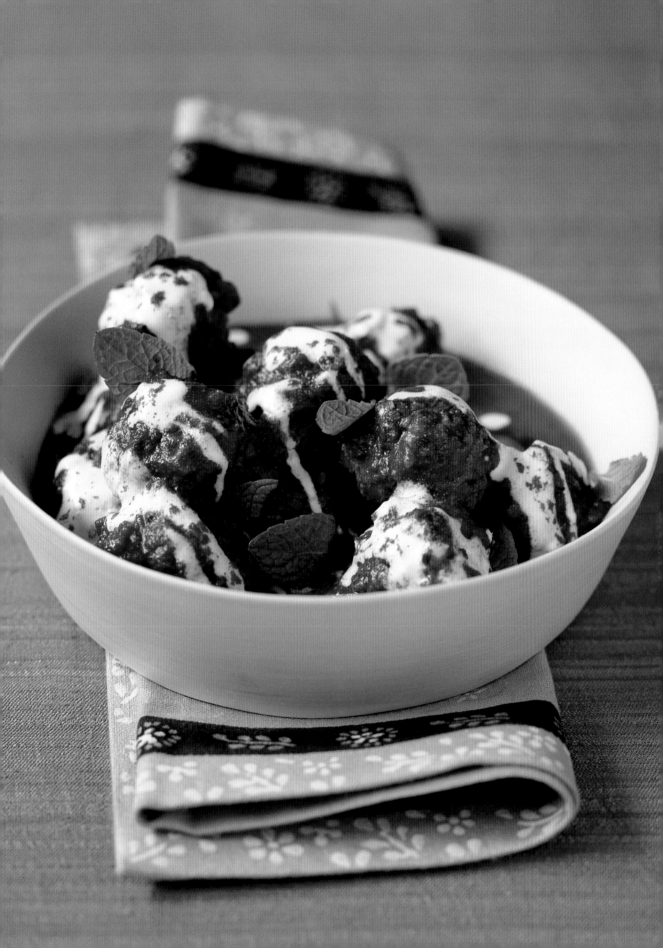

KHEEMA MUTTER

A staple northern Indian dish, this versatile, spiced beef mince with peas is flavoured with fragrant coriander, aromatic garlic, spicy green chillies and juicy, fresh tomatoes. If you fancy a change, you can also try cooking this dish using a mixture of chicken and pork mince.

SERVES 4 ❄

Syns per serving
Original: 1½

EASY

Preparation time 15 minutes
Cooking time 30 minutes

Fry Light

2 garlic cloves, peeled and crushed

2 fresh green chillies, deseeded and chopped

2 tsp ground coriander

2 tsp ground cumin

500g/1lb 2oz extra-lean minced beef

150g/5oz frozen peas

2 tbsp medium curry powder

3 tbsp tomato purée

4 ripe tomatoes, finely chopped

¼ tsp artificial sweetener

250ml/9fl oz hot beef stock made with Bovril

salt

2 tbsp very low fat natural yogurt

a large handful of freshly chopped coriander leaves

1. Spray a large frying pan with Fry Light and place over a medium heat. Add the garlic, chillies, ground coriander, cumin and minced beef and stir-fry for 6–7 minutes or until the meat is sealed and browned.

2. Stir in the peas, curry powder, tomato purée, chopped tomatoes and sweetener. Stir and cook for 3–4 minutes and then add the hot stock. Bring to the boil, cover, reduce the heat and simmer gently for 8–10 minutes, stirring occasionally.

3. Remove from the heat, season with salt, stir in the yogurt and chopped coriander and serve.

TIP If you like your food hot, leave the seeds in the chillies!

BEEF MADRAS

HOT 🌶🌶🌶

Madras curries originate from the east coast of southern India and are usually very spicy and robust in flavour – not for the faint-hearted! This recipe uses lean beef, but you can use lamb if you prefer.

SERVES 4 ❄
Syns per serving
Original: Free
EASY
Preparation time 15 minutes
Cooking time 1 hour 45 minutes

Fry Light

1 onion, peeled and finely chopped

4 cloves

6 green cardamom pods

2 fresh red chillies, finely chopped

1 tsp peeled and finely grated ginger

2 garlic cloves, peeled and crushed

2 dried red chillies

1 tbsp Madras curry powder

900g/2lb beef fillets, all visible fat removed, cut into bite-sized chunks

2 tsp ground coriander

1 tsp ground cumin

250ml/9fl oz beef stock made with Bovril

salt

TO SERVE
freshly chopped coriander leaves

1. Spray a saucepan liberally with Fry Light and place over a medium heat. Add the onion, cloves and cardamom and stir-fry for 3–4 minutes.

2. Add the fresh chilli, ginger, garlic and dried chilli and stir-fry for a further 2 minutes.

3. Add the curry powder and beef chunks to the saucepan and stir-fry for 6–8 minutes until the meat is sealed. Add the ground coriander, cumin and stock and bring to the boil. Season with salt, cover tightly and reduce the heat to low. Cook gently for 1½ hours, stirring occasionally, until the meat is tender. Remove the pan from the heat and scatter over some chopped coriander before serving.

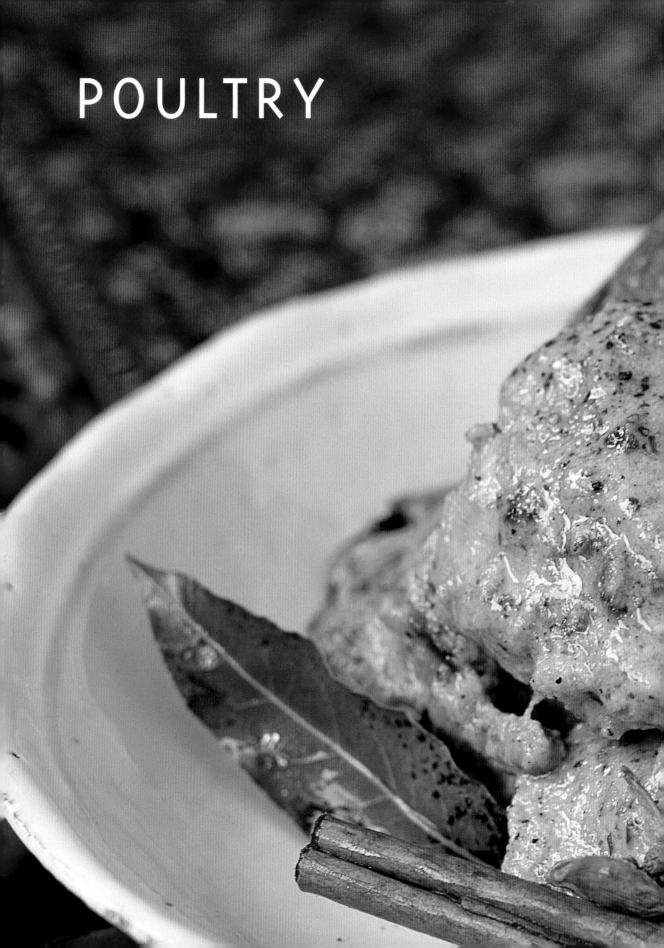

POULTRY

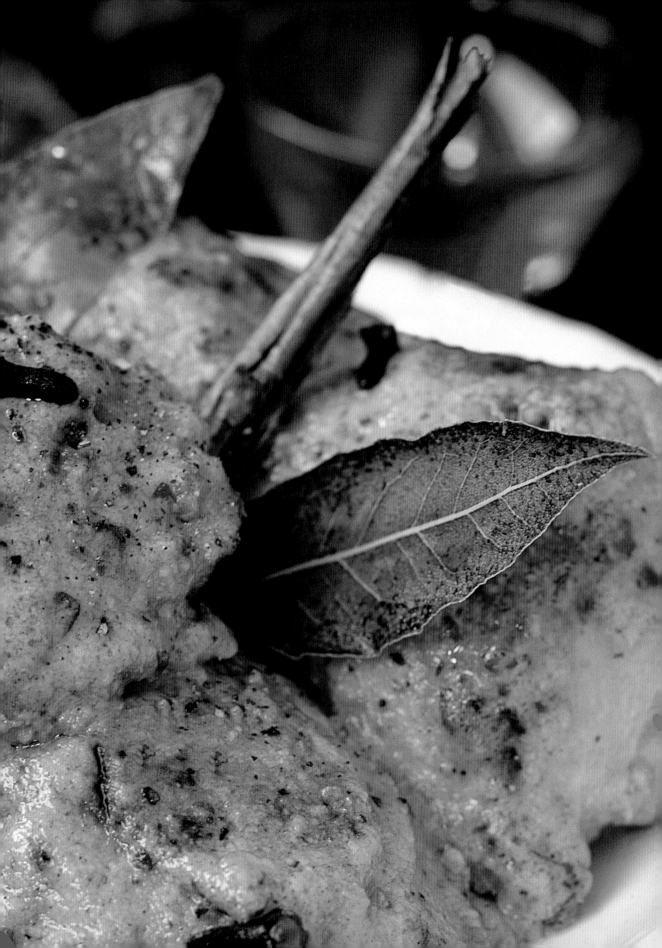

ANDHRA CHILLI CHICKEN

VERY HOT ⁄⁄⁄⁄

Originating from the region of Andhra Pradesh in southern India, this curry is really fiery but delicious if you have a high threshold for hot, hot food!

SERVES 4 ❅
Syns per serving
Original: ½
EASY
Preparation time 10 minutes
Cooking time 1 hour

3 tbsp tomato purée
2 garlic cloves, peeled and crushed
2 fresh red chillies, deseeded and chopped
5 dried red chillies
1 tsp sea salt
¼ tsp artificial sweetener
1 tsp hot chilli powder
1 tsp paprika
1 tbsp medium curry powder
Fry Light
1 tsp cumin seeds
1 onion, peeled and finely grated
3–4 fresh curry leaves
1 tsp ground coriander
1 tsp ground cumin
400g can chopped tomatoes
250ml/9fl oz chicken stock made with Bovril
8 chicken thighs, skinless
salt

1. Place the tomato purée, garlic, fresh and dried chillies, salt, sweetener, chilli powder, paprika and curry powder in a food processor, add 60ml/2fl oz of water and blend until smooth. Set aside until needed.

2. Spray a large saucepan with Fry Light and place over a medium heat. Add the cumin seeds and fry for 1 minute before adding the onion and curry leaves and cooking for a further 4–5 minutes.

3. Add the chilli paste mixture and fry for 2–3 minutes. Stir in the coriander and cumin, tomatoes, stock and chicken and bring to the boil. Cover, reduce the heat to low and cook gently for 35–45 minutes or until the chicken is tender, stirring occasionally. Season to taste and serve immediately.

CREAMY CHICKEN CURRY

MEDIUM

Deliciously creamy and with just the right amount of heat, this is a curry that's too good to hurry!

SERVES 4 ✳

Syns per serving
Original: Free

EASY
Preparation time 15 minutes
Cooking time 15 minutes

salt and freshly ground black pepper

4 x 150g/5oz chicken breasts, skinless

Fry Light

3 garlic cloves, peeled and crushed

½ tsp each crushed cardamom seeds and ground turmeric

1 tbsp ground coriander

1 tsp each ground ginger and cumin

1-2 tsp mild or medium chilli powder

1 tbsp tomato purée

1 onion, peeled and grated

100g pot very low fat natural fromage frais

1 tbsp freshly chopped coriander

TO SERVE
freshly chopped coriander leaves
lemon wedges

1. Season the chicken and lightly spray with Fry Light. Place under a hot grill and cook for 6–8 minutes on each side or until cooked through. Remove from the grill and cut into bite-sized pieces.

2. Spray a pan with Fry Light and heat until hot. Add the garlic, cardamom, turmeric, coriander, ginger, cumin and chilli powder and fry for 1 minute. Add the tomato purée and grated onion and continue frying for a further 3–4 minutes.

3. Add the chicken to the pan along with 150ml/5fl oz of water and cook for 5–6 minutes. Stir in the fromage frais, season to taste and gently heat through. When hot, remove from the heat and stir in the chopped coriander. Serve immediately garnished with freshly chopped coriander and a few lemon wedges.

CLASSIC CHICKEN CURRY

This classic dish is cooked the length and breadth of India with a few variations – but basically it is a wonderful stew of chicken cooked with tomatoes and spices and will perk up any jaded palate.

SERVES 4 ✳

Syns per serving
Original: Free

WORTH THE EFFORT
Preparation time 10 minutes
Cooking time 1 hour

1kg/2lb 4oz chicken thighs, skinless and boneless, cut into large pieces

salt and freshly ground black pepper

Fry Light

1 onion, peeled and finely chopped

2 tsp peeled and finely grated ginger

2 tsp crushed garlic

1 tsp ground cumin

1 tsp ground coriander

½ tsp crushed cardamom seeds

¼ tsp ground cloves

1 tsp ground cinnamon

1 tbsp mild or medium curry powder

1 tsp paprika

¼ tsp turmeric

400g can chopped tomatoes

300ml/½pt chicken stock made with Bovril

¼ tsp artificial sweetener

TO SERVE
freshly chopped coriander leaves
sliced fresh green chillies

1. Place the chicken on a plate, season well and set aside.

2. Spray a frying pan with Fry Light and place over a medium heat. Add the onion and stir-fry for 5–6 minutes or until starting to lightly brown.

3. Stir in the ginger, garlic, cumin, coriander, cardamom, cloves, cinnamon, curry powder, paprika and turmeric and stir-fry over a high heat for 1–2 minutes.

4. Add the chicken and cook for 2–3 minutes until sealed, then add the tomatoes, stock and sweetener. Bring to the boil, cover tightly, reduce the heat to low and allow to simmer gently for 40–45 minutes, stirring occasionally until the chicken is cooked through.

5. Remove the frying pan from the heat, adjust the seasoning to taste and serve garnished with freshly chopped coriander and sliced green chillies.

TIP Create your own spice mix if you prefer – grind all your favourite spices together and place in a pepper mill so you have a great blend ready to use whenever you want.

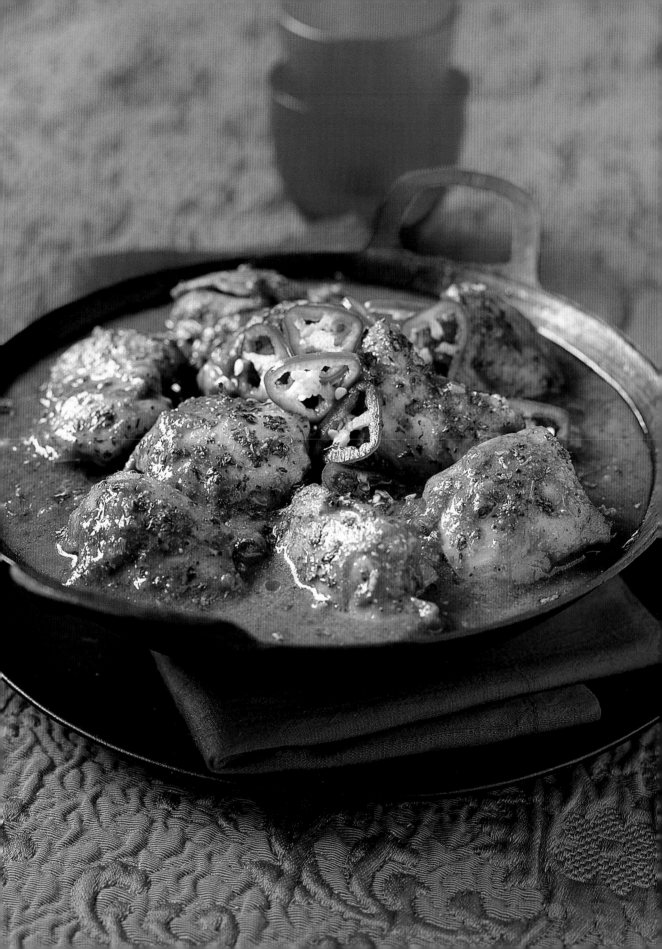

BALTI CHICKEN

The emergence of Balti cooking originated in Birmingham and not India as you would expect! However, it is a cooking style that is here to stay and a major part of the Indian, Pakistani and British communities. The word 'Balti' actually means a metal bucket but over here it is taken to mean a karahi or wok in which the dish is cooked.

SERVES 4 ✱
Syns per serving
Original: Free
EASY
Preparation time 15 minutes
Cooking time 25 minutes

Fry Light

2 onions, peeled and thinly sliced

2 fresh red chillies, deseeded and thinly sliced

6–8 fresh curry leaves

3 garlic cloves, peeled and crushed

1 tsp peeled and finely grated ginger

1 tbsp ground coriander

2 tsp medium curry powder

500g/1lb 2oz lean minced chicken

juice of 1 lemon

a small handful of freshly chopped mint leaves

a small handful of freshly chopped coriander leaves

salt

1. Spray a large frying pan or wok with Fry Light and place over a medium heat. Add the onion, chilli and curry leaves and stir-fry for 4–5 minutes. Add 4 tablespoons of water and continue to stir-fry for 2–3 minutes.

2. Add the garlic, ginger, coriander, curry powder and chicken mince and stir-fry over a high heat for 6–8 minutes. Add 5 tablespoons of water and continue to stir-fry for 3–4 minutes or until the chicken is sealed and cooked through.

3. Remove from the heat and stir in the lemon juice and freshly chopped mint and coriander. Season with salt and serve immediately.

CHICKEN GHASSI

MEDIUM

This curry originates from Mangalore on the coast of western India and uses coconut milk, which is used in many dishes in this region. Here we've used reduced-fat coconut milk to keep the taste and reduce the Syns.

SERVES 4
Syns per serving
Original: 3
EASY
Preparation time 10 minutes
Cooking time 40 minutes

Fry Light

1 large onion, peeled and finely grated

4 chicken breasts, skinless and boneless, cut into bite-sized pieces

1 tsp garam masala

1 tsp peeled and finely grated ginger

2 garlic cloves, peeled and crushed

1–2 tsp mild or medium chilli powder

¼ tsp turmeric

250ml/9fl oz chicken stock made with Bovril

200ml/7fl oz reduced-fat coconut milk

salt

1. Spray a frying pan with Fry Light and place over a medium heat. Add the onion and stir-fry for 8–10 minutes or until it starts to lightly brown.

2. Add the chicken and continue to fry for 4–5 minutes, stirring occasionally, before mixing in the garam masala, ginger, garlic, chilli powder and turmeric.

3. Pour over the stock and coconut milk, bring to the boil, season with salt, cover tightly and reduce the heat to low. Simmer gently for 20–25 minutes, stirring occasionally until the chicken is cooked through. Serve immediately.

MALAI CHICKEN

In this very simple to cook chicken dish, originally made with cream, hence its name malai, *chicken pieces are cooked with just a few spices. As an alternative to the cream, we've used very low fat natural yogurt.*

SERVES 4
Syns per serving
Original: Free

EASY
Preparation time 5–6 minutes
Cooking time 20–25 minutes

Fry Light

1 tsp crushed cardamom seeds

2 tsp mild curry powder

700g/1lb 8oz chicken breasts, skinless and boneless, cut into bite-sized pieces

1 tsp mild chilli powder

½ tsp turmeric

salt and freshly ground black pepper

1 tbsp tomato purée

150g pot very low fat natural yogurt

150ml/5fl oz chicken stock made with Bovril

1. Spray a saucepan with Fry Light and place over a medium heat. Add the cardamom and curry powder and stir-fry for 10–15 seconds.

2. Throw in the chicken and fry on a high heat for 5–6 minutes. Add the chilli powder and turmeric and season well.

3. Mix together the tomato purée, yogurt and stock and pour into the pan, bring to a simmer, cover and cook gently for 15 minutes or until tender (do not boil or the mixture will curdle). Stir well, remove from the heat and serve drizzled with a little more yogurt if liked.

SILKEN CHICKEN

In this delicious recipe of tender, silken chicken (hence its name), chicken breasts are marinated with spices and yogurt and then baked to perfection.

SERVES 4 ❄

Syns per serving
Original: Free

EASY

Preparation time 15 minutes
(plus standing and chilling)
Cooking time 15 minutes

4 chicken breasts, skinless

salt and freshly ground black pepper

2 tbsp lemon juice

4 tbsp very low fat natural yogurt

1 garlic clove, peeled and crushed

1 tsp peeled and finely grated ginger

1½ tsp garam masala

1½ tsp mild chilli powder

1½ tsp ground cumin

2 tsp dried mint

1. Place the chicken on a work surface and make 3–4 diagonal cuts across the top of each breast. Arrange the chicken in a single layer in a shallow container and season liberally. Squeeze over the lemon juice, toss to coat well and allow to stand for 5–10 minutes.

2. Mix together the yogurt, garlic, ginger and 1 tsp each of garam masala, chilli powder and cumin. Pour over the chicken to coat evenly, cover and chill in the fridge overnight to let the flavours penetrate.

3. Preheat the oven to 220°C/Gas 7. Remove the chicken from the fridge and place on a non-stick baking sheet. Sprinkle over the remaining garam masala, chilli powder and cumin along with the dried mint. Season well and bake for 12–15 minutes or until tender and cooked through. Serve immediately.

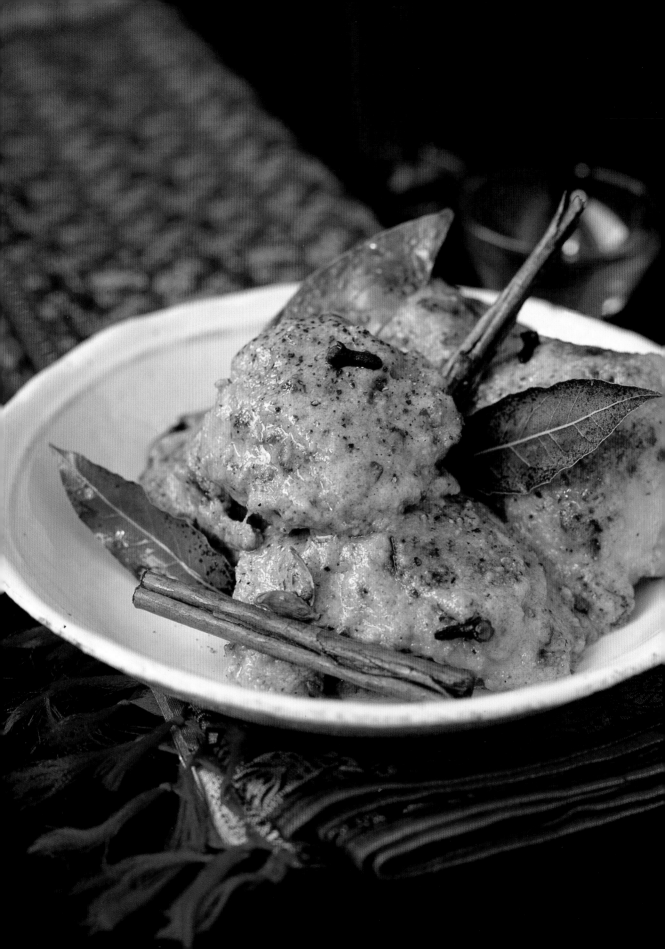

SHAHI MURGH

This chicken dish, also know as Royal Chicken, was once served in the royal Mughal palaces of India. Cooked in yogurt with spices, it is a straightforward yet delicious dish.

SERVES 4 ❋
Syns per serving
Original: Free
EASY
Preparation time 10 minutes
Cooking time 50 minutes
(plus standing)

salt and freshly ground black
pepper

1kg/2lb 4oz chicken thighs,
skinless

250g/9oz very low fat natural
yogurt

2 tsp ground cumin

2 tsp ground coriander

¼ tsp mild chilli powder

5 tbsp freshly chopped coriander

Fry Light

10 cardamom pods

8 cloves

2 cinnamon sticks

3 bay leaves

1. Season the chicken and set aside. Place the yogurt in a bowl and lightly beat until smooth. Season with salt and pepper, then add the cumin, ground coriander, chilli powder and chopped coriander, mix well and set aside.

2. Spray a large frying pan liberally with Fry Light and place over a high heat. Add the cardamom, cloves, cinnamon and bay leaves and fry for 1–2 minutes. Add the chicken in a single layer and brown both sides. Pour over the yogurt mixture, stir well, turn the heat to low, cover tightly and simmer gently for 20–25 minutes, stirring occasionally.

3. Uncover and cook for a further 3–4 minutes until the sauce thickens and clings to the chicken. Remove from the heat and allow to stand for 5 minutes before serving.

CHICKEN KAUKSWE

This is a popular Burmese curry. It is traditionally served with egg noodles and lots of accompaniments for people to help themselves to at the table – making it a great entertaining dish.

SERVES 4 ❋
Syns per serving
Original: 3

WORTH THE EFFORT
Preparation time 10 minutes
Cooking time 1 hour

5 garlic cloves, peeled and chopped

2 onions, peeled and grated

1 tbsp peeled and finely grated ginger

1–2 fresh red chillies, deseeded and chopped

Fry Light

450g/1lb chicken breasts, skinless and boneless, cut into thin strips

350ml/12fl oz passata

200ml/7fl oz chicken stock made with Bovril

200ml/7fl oz reduced-fat coconut milk

salt

TO SERVE
hard-boiled eggs, finely chopped

spring onions, trimmed and finely sliced

freshly chopped coriander leaves

1. Place the garlic, onion, ginger and chilli in a food processor and blend until fairly well combined.

2. Spray a frying pan with Fry Light and place over a high heat. Add the blended mixture and stir-fry for 4–5 minutes.

3. Add the chicken strips and stir-fry for 5–6 minutes before pouring the passata and stock over the top. Bring to the boil, cover, reduce the heat to low and cook gently for 30 minutes. Uncover, add the coconut milk and continue to cook gently for 10–15 minutes. Season with salt and remove from the heat.

4. Serve as it is or ladle over boiled noodles (1½ Syns per 25g/1oz) and top with a selection of the accompaniments listed below.

TIP This dish also works well accompanied with finely chopped mint or dill, cucumber, carrot and radish.

TANDOORI SPATCHCOCK POUSSIN

MILD ✦

The national dish of India, Tandoori chicken, is enjoyed by all. Usually the use of red food colour in the marinade makes the typical restaurant version of this dish very, very red in colour – and to me a little bit scary! Here I have used spatchcock poussin, but if you prefer, you could use six chicken thigh joints instead.

SERVES 4 ❄
Syns per serving
Original: Free
EASY
Preparation time 15 minutes
(plus chilling)
Cooking time 20–25 minutes

2 spatchcock poussins, skinless
250g/9oz very low fat natural yogurt
1 tbsp tomato purée
1 tsp peeled and finely grated ginger
5 garlic cloves, peeled and crushed
2 tsp ground cumin
2 tsp ground coriander
½ small onion, peeled and roughly chopped
1 tbsp mild paprika
salt and freshly ground black pepper
1 tsp garam masala
1 tsp cayenne pepper
1 tsp amchoor (dried mango powder) (optional)

TO SERVE
lemon wedges
freshly chopped coriander leaves

1. Place the spatchcock poussins in a dish and, using a sharp knife, make little cuts all over the flesh (this will allow the marinade to penetrate).

2. Place the yogurt, tomato purée, ginger, garlic, cumin, coriander, onion and paprika in a food processor and blend until smooth. Season well, pour over the poussins and rub in well. Cover and chill in the fridge overnight to let the flavours penetrate.

3. When ready to cook, remove the poussins from the fridge and preheat the oven to 200°C/Gas 6. Place the poussins on a non-stick baking sheet and sprinkle over the garam masala, cayenne pepper and amchoor (if using). Bake for 20–25 minutes or until cooked through. Serve immediately with lemon wedges and coriander leaves to garnish.

TIP Amchoor can be bought in large supermarkets or Asian green-grocers. If you can't find it, use lime or lemon juice as a substitute.

CREAMY CHICKEN KORMA

This favourite dish is well liked by all for its mild, yet fragrant flavour. The original recipe uses cream, but here we use very low fat fromage frais to give the same effect without the Syns!

SERVES 4 ❄
Syns per serving
Original: Free
EASY
Preparation time 10 minutes
Cooking time 35 minutes

Fry Light

3 bay leaves

1 cinnamon stick

1 tsp crushed cardamom seeds

¼ tsp crushed cloves

2 tsp cumin seeds

1 onion, peeled and finely grated

1 tbsp ground coriander

1 tbsp ground cumin

3 tsp peeled and finely grated ginger

3 tsp peeled and finely crushed garlic

200g can chopped tomatoes

2 tsp korma curry powder

1kg/2lb 4oz chicken breasts, skinless and boneless, cut into bite-sized pieces

200ml/7fl oz chicken stock made with Bovril

salt and freshly ground black pepper

5 tbsp very low fat natural fromage frais

TO SERVE
freshly chopped mint leaves

1. Spray a large frying pan with Fry Light and place over a high heat. Add the bay leaves, cinnamon, cardamom seeds, cloves, cumin seeds and onion and stir-fry for 5–6 minutes.

2. Add the coriander, cumin, ginger, garlic, tomatoes and korma curry powder and stir-fry for another 3–4 minutes.

3. Throw the chicken into the pan and pour over the stock. Bring to the boil, season well, cover tightly, reduce the heat to low and allow to simmer gently for 20–25 minutes, stirring occasionally.

4. Remove the pan from the heat and stir in the fromage frais. Serve immediately garnished with mint.

CHICKEN TIKKA MASALA

MEDIUM 🌶🌶

*Here is another Indian dish that has its origins in England. It started its life as chicken tikka – which is marinated meat pieces (*tikka *literally means pieces). In the Indian restaurants in England, they add a creamy spiced sauce to it and, hey presto, it has become one of the nation's most popular dishes.*

SERVES 4 ✷
Syns per serving
Original: ½
EASY
Preparation time 10 minutes
(plus marinating)
Cooking time 40 minutes

700g/1lb 8oz chicken breast fillets, skinless and cut into bite-sized pieces

4 tbsp tikka masala powder

110g/4oz very low fat natural yogurt

salt and freshly ground black pepper

Fry Light

1 small onion, peeled and finely grated

4 garlic cloves, peeled and crushed

1 tsp peeled and finely grated ginger

1 fresh red chilli, deseeded and finely chopped

2 tbsp tomato purée

¼ tsp artificial sweetener

5 tbsp very low fat natural fromage frais

1. Place the chicken pieces in a bowl. Mix half of the tikka masala powder into the yogurt. Season well and pour over the chicken. Toss to coat well, cover and marinate in the fridge overnight.

2. Spray a frying pan with Fry Light and place over a medium-high heat. Add the onion and stir-fry continuously for 5–6 minutes. Add the garlic, ginger, red chilli and remaining tikka masala powder and stir-fry for 2–3 minutes. Stir in the tomato purée and sweetener along with 250ml/9fl oz of water and bring to the boil. Reduce the heat and cook gently for 12–15 minutes, stirring often. Remove from the heat, season well and then stir in the fromage frais and keep warm.

3. Remove the chicken from the fridge and thread onto 8 metal skewers. Spray lightly with Fry Light and cook under a medium-hot grill for 12–15 minutes, turning once or twice, until cooked through. Remove the chicken pieces from the skewers, stir into the sauce and serve.

JALFREZI CHICKEN

Another restaurant favourite, a jalfrezi is a stir-fry curry cooked with mixed peppers, onions and spices. You could use strips of lean beef, pork or lamb as a substitute for the chicken if liked.

SERVES 4 ❄

Syns per serving
Original: Free

EASY

Preparation time 15 minutes
Cooking time 30 minutes

4 chicken breast fillets, skinless
Fry Light
1 tsp cumin seeds
1 onion, peeled and finely sliced
1 red pepper, deseeded and thinly sliced
1 yellow pepper, deseeded and thinly sliced
2 garlic cloves, peeled and crushed
1 tsp peeled and finely grated ginger
1 tbsp medium curry powder
½ tsp mild or medium chilli powder
1 tsp ground cumin
1 tsp ground coriander
salt and freshly ground black pepper
400g can chopped tomatoes
a large handful of chopped coriander leaves

TO SERVE

very low fat natural yogurt
chopped cucumber

1. Place the chicken breasts between sheets of cling film and flatten with a rolling pin. Remove the cling film, cut the chicken into thin strips and set aside.

2. Spray a large frying pan with Fry Light, place over a medium heat, add the cumin seeds and stir-fry for 1–2 minutes. Add the onion, peppers, garlic and ginger and fry for a further 6–8 minutes.

3. Add the curry powder, chilli powder, cumin and coriander. Season well and fry for 1–2 minutes.

4. Throw in the chicken, increase the heat to high and stir-fry for 4–5 minutes. Stir in the tomatoes and coriander along with 100ml/3½fl oz of water. Cover, reduce the heat to low and cook gently for about 15 minutes or until the chicken is tender. Remove from the heat, adjust the seasoning to taste and serve immediately with a bowl of very low fat natural yogurt and chopped cucumber.

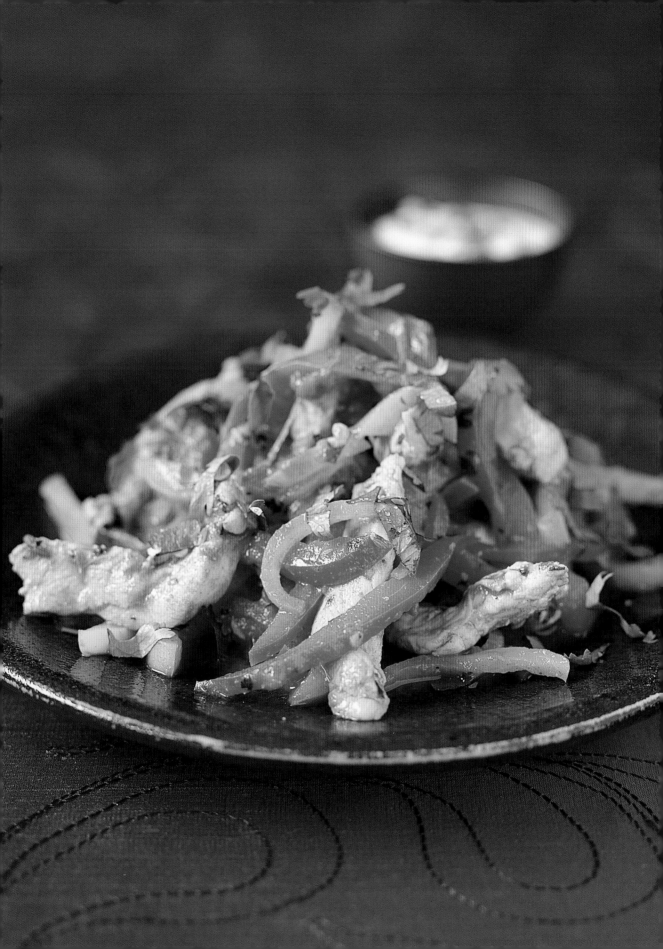

CHICKEN DOPIAZA

Literally translated, dopiaza *means 'two onions', but the dish really uses a lot of onions and shallots. It is cooked gently for the sweetness of the onions to come through.*

SERVES 4 ❄
Syns per serving
Original: Free
EASY
Preparation time 15 minutes
Cooking time 1 hour 15 minutes

Fry Light

8 shallots, peeled and halved

2 bay leaves

10 cardamom pods

6 cloves

3 dried red chillies

8 black peppercorns

2 onions, peeled and finely grated

3 garlic cloves, peeled and crushed

1 tsp peeled and finely grated ginger

1 tsp ground coriander

1 tsp ground cumin

¼ tsp turmeric

salt

6 ripe plum tomatoes, roughly chopped

350ml/12fl oz chicken stock made with Bovril

8 chicken thighs (drumsticks will also work well), on the bone, skinless

1. Spray a large saucepan with Fry Light and place over a medium heat. Add the shallots and stir-fry for 6–7 minutes until lightly browned. Remove from the pan and set aside.

2. Lightly spray the pan with Fry Light again and place over a medium heat. When hot, add the bay leaves, cardamom pods, cloves, dried chillies and peppercorns and fry for 2–3 minutes. Add the onion, garlic, ginger, coriander, cumin and turmeric, season with salt and cook for 4–5 minutes, stirring often.

3. Stir in the tomatoes, shallots and stock and bring to the boil. Add the chicken thighs, cover tightly, reduce the heat to low and cook gently for about an hour or until the chicken is meltingly tender. Remove from the heat and serve.

BOMBAY GREEN CHICKEN CURRY

MEDIUM 🌶🌶

This chicken curry was always made in my house on a Sunday for lunch with family and friends. It is fresh and flavourful and tastes even better the next day – if there are any leftovers!

SERVES 4 ❄
Syns per serving
Original: 3
WORTH THE EFFORT
Preparation time 15 minutes
Cooking time 35–40 minutes

Fry Light

1 onion, peeled and finely grated

4 garlic cloves, peeled and crushed

2 tsp peeled and finely grated ginger

a large handful of freshly chopped coriander leaves

4 tbsp freshly chopped mint leaves

2 fresh green chillies, deseeded and chopped

¼ tsp crushed cardamom seeds

1 tbsp ground cumin

½ tsp ground cinnamon

1 tbsp ground coriander

¼ tsp artificial sweetener

200ml/7fl oz reduced-fat coconut milk

700g/1lb 8oz chicken thighs, skinless and boneless, cut into bite-sized pieces

400ml/14fl oz chicken stock made with Bovril

salt and freshly ground black pepper

1. Spray a large frying pan with Fry Light and place over a medium heat. Add the onion to the pan and stir-fry for 4–5 minutes or until it starts to lightly brown.

2. Meanwhile place the garlic, ginger, fresh coriander, mint, green chilli, cardamom, cumin, cinnamon, coriander and sweetener in a food processor and blend until combined. Add the coconut milk to the food processor and continue to blend until the whole mixture is fairly smooth.

3. Add the chicken to the onion and continue to fry over a high heat for 5–6 minutes. Add the stock and the coconut mixture, season well, bring to the boil, cover tightly, reduce the heat to low and cook gently for 20–25 minutes, stirring occasionally, until the chicken is tender and cooked through. Remove from the heat and serve immediately.

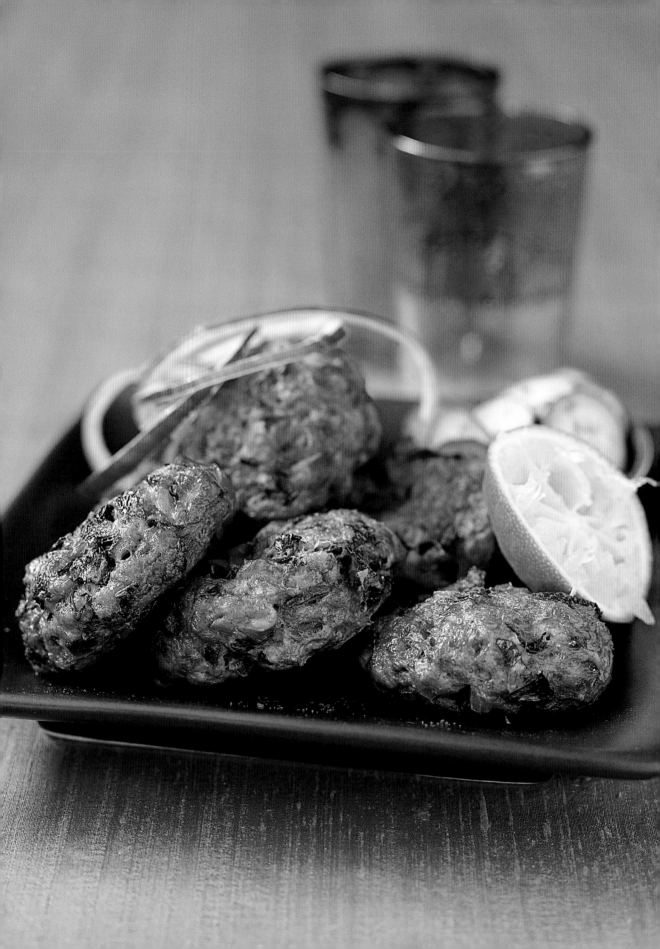

TURKEY SHAMI KEBABS

MEDIUM ⁑

Usually made from minced lamb or beef, these kebabs are lightly spiced. Originally cooked in a clay oven or tandoor, here they are simply baked in a hot oven. Serve with steamed vegetables or a large salad for a great meal.

SERVES 4 ❆
Syns per serving
Original: Free
EASY
Preparation time 15 minutes
(plus chilling)
Cooking time 20 minutes

800g/1lb 12oz lean minced
turkey

1 small red onion, peeled and
finely grated

1 tsp peeled and finely grated
ginger

1 tbsp medium curry powder

1 tsp finely grated lime zest

1 fresh red chilli, deseeded and
finely chopped

3 tbsp freshly chopped coriander
leaves

2 tbsp freshly chopped mint
leaves

2 tbsp very low fat natural
yogurt

salt and freshly ground black
pepper

Fry Light

TO SERVE
red onion rings
lime wedges

1. Place the turkey in a mixing bowl with the onion, ginger, curry powder, lime zest, chilli, coriander, mint and yogurt. Season well and, using your hands, mix until well combined. Cover and chill in the fridge for 6–8 hours (overnight if possible) to allow the flavours to develop.

2. Preheat the oven to 200°C/Gas 6. Divide the turkey mixture into 12 portions and shape each portion into a flat, oval kebab shape. Place on a baking sheet lined with baking parchment and spray with Fry Light. Bake for 15–20 minutes until lightly browned and cooked through. Remove from the oven and serve with red onion rings and lime wedges to squeeze over.

SAAG WALLA TURKEY

In this delicious and healthy dish, turkey pieces are cooked in a creamy, spiced spinach sauce. You can use chicken instead of turkey if you wish – they both taste great!

SERVES 4
Syns per serving
Original: Free
EASY
Preparation time 10 minutes
Cooking time 50 minutes

1kg/2lb 4oz turkey breasts, skinless and boneless, cut into bite-sized pieces

5 tbsp very low fat natural yogurt

2 tsp garam masala

3 tsp peeled and finely grated ginger

7 garlic cloves, peeled and crushed

1 tbsp ground coriander

450g/1lb frozen spinach, defrosted

salt and freshly ground black pepper

Fry Light

1 onion, peeled and finely chopped

2 tsp cumin seeds

2 fresh green chillies, deseeded and chopped

juice of 1 lemon

1. Place the turkey in a bowl. Mix together the yogurt, 1 tsp garam masala, 1 tsp ginger, 2 cloves crushed garlic and the ground coriander and rub all over the turkey pieces to coat evenly. Cover and chill in the fridge for 4–5 hours, or overnight if time permits, to allow the flavours to develop.

2. Place the spinach in a saucepan, season well and wilt for 6–8 minutes over a medium heat. Remove from the heat, transfer to a food processor and blend to a purée.

3. Meanwhile, spray a frying pan with Fry Light and place over a medium heat. Add the onion and stir-fry for 10 minutes or until it starts to brown. Stir in the cumin seeds, green chilli, remaining garam masala, ginger and garlic and continue to fry for 3–4 minutes.

4. Increase the heat to high, add the turkey and fry for 4–5 minutes. Stir in the spinach purée, bring to the boil, cover tightly, reduce the heat to low and simmer gently for 15–20 minutes or until cooked through.

5. Uncover the pan, season well and cook on a high heat for 2–3 minutes. Remove from the heat and squeeze over the lemon juice before serving with Sukki gobi (see page 192).

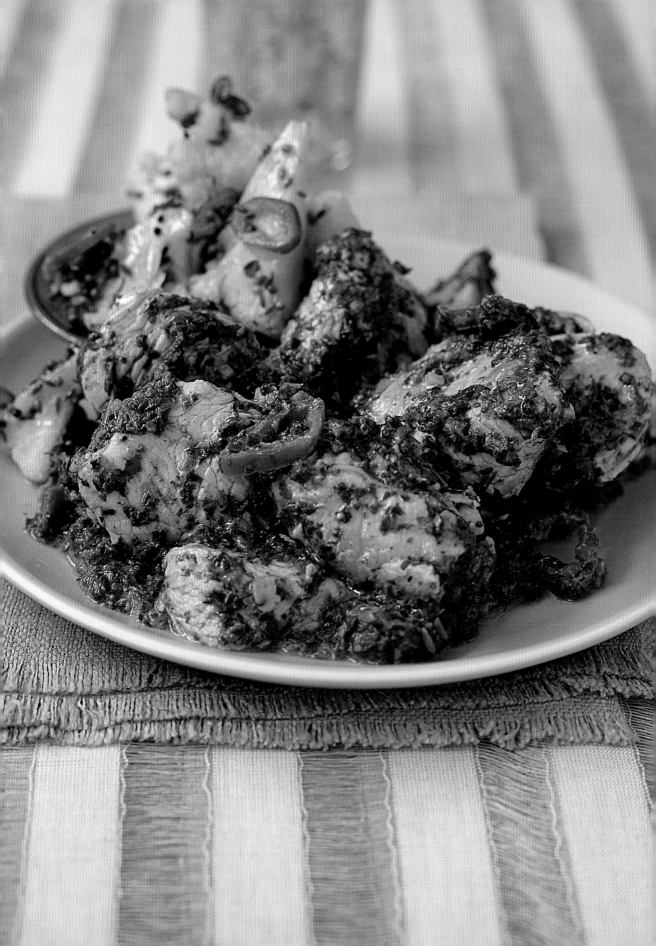

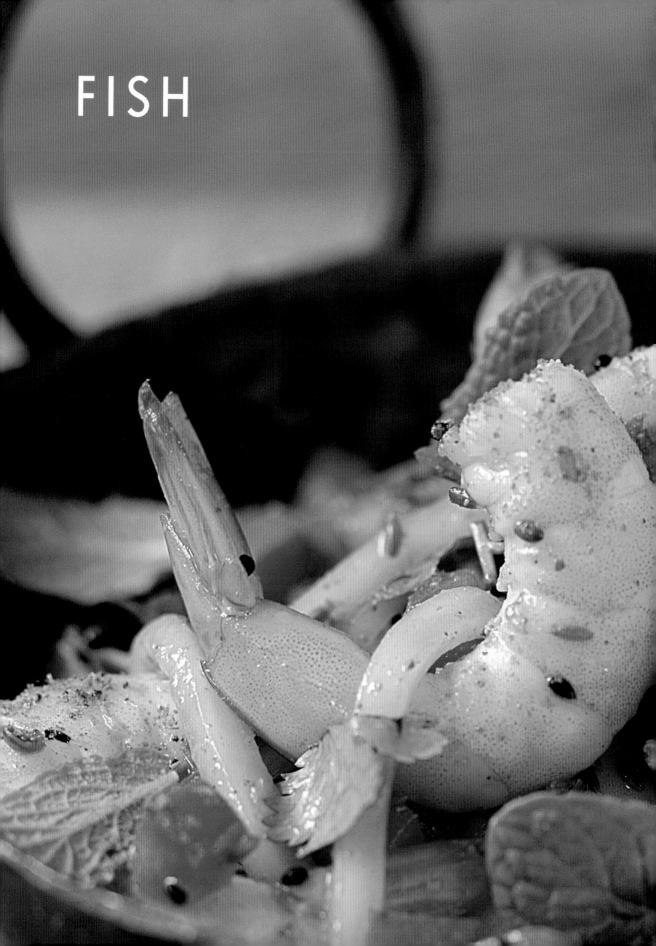

FISH

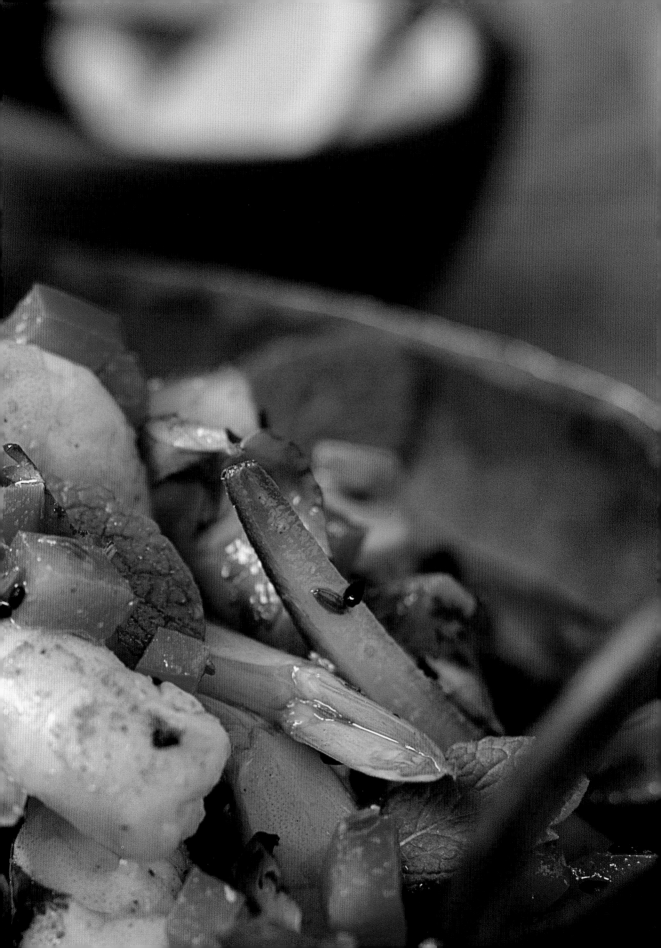

KONKAN-STYLE MUSSELS

The western Konkan coast of India is teeming with fresh seafood. In this recipe, fresh mussels are steamed with a rich blend of warming spices. Always make sure the mussels are absolutely fresh – use a good fishmonger or supermarket when buying them.

SERVES 4
Syns per serving
Original: 2
EASY
Preparation time 5 minutes
Cooking time 15 minutes

Fry Light

2 shallots, peeled and very finely chopped

1 fresh red chilli, cut lengthways and deseeded

3cm/1¼in piece of ginger, peeled and cut into thin shreds

2 garlic cloves, peeled and cut into thin shreds

2 plum tomatoes, finely chopped

1 tbsp medium or hot curry powder

600g/1lb 6oz fresh mussels

a large handful of chopped coriander leaves

3 tbsp grated fresh coconut (optional)

1. Spray a large wok or saucepan with Fry Light and place over a medium heat. Add the shallots, red chilli, ginger and garlic and stir-fry for 3–4 minutes. Stir in the tomatoes, curry powder and 200ml/7fl oz of water and continue to cook over a high heat for 4–5 minutes.

2. Tip in the mussels, stir to mix and cover tightly. Continue to cook over a high heat for 6–8 minutes or until the mussels have opened, discarding any that remain closed.

3. Stir in the chopped coriander and sprinkle over the grated coconut (if using) and serve immediately with a fresh salad or steamed vegetables of your choice.

LAL MASALA BHANGDA

The word masala *simply means a 'spice mixture'. You can have many different combinations and textures of masalas from dry mixtures to wet pastes. Here we use a wet masala paste made with red chillies and spices to spread over the fish before grilling. You could use any firm fish fillet for this recipe if desired.*

SERVES 4 ❄
Syns per serving
Original: ½

EXTRA EASY
Preparation time 10 minutes
Cooking time 10 minutes

4 large mackerel, each around 300g/11oz, cleaned and gutted

juice of 3 large limes

2 fresh red chillies, deseeded and very finely chopped

1 tsp hot chilli powder

2 tsp peeled and finely grated ginger

2 tsp peeled and finely grated garlic

1 tbsp mild curry powder

1 tsp ground cumin

1 tsp ground coriander

4 tbsp tomato purée

¼ tsp artificial sweetener

1 tbsp vinegar

salt

1. Place the fish on a clean work surface and make 4–5 deep diagonal cuts on each side of the fish.

2. Make the masala paste by combining all the remaining ingredients, except the salt, in a food processor (or by using a pestle and mortar) with a few tablespoons of water and blend until fairly smooth. Season well and spread this mixture over the fish, rubbing it into the cuts on either side.

3. Place the fish under a preheated grill for 6–8 minutes on each side until thoroughly cooked and lightly charred at the edges. Serve immediately.

CHILLI-SPICED SQUID

HOT ///

Always try to get fresh squid from the fishmonger for this dish. You can use frozen but make sure that it is properly defrosted before you cook it. When cooking squid it is important to remember that it only needs a very short time. Longer cooking will leave it rubbery in texture.

SERVES 4 ❄

Syns per serving
Original: Free

WORTH THE EFFORT
Preparation time 10 minutes
(plus standing)
Cooking time 20 minutes

700g/1lb 8oz fresh squid, cleaned and cut into bite-sized rings or pieces

2 tsp sea salt

juice of 2 lemons

1 tsp ground coriander

1 tsp ground cumin

1 tsp hot chilli powder

1 tsp tomato purée

1 fresh red chilli, deseeded and finely sliced

1 tsp peeled and finely grated ginger

1 clove garlic, peeled and crushed

Fry Light

a large handful of chopped coriander leaves

1 small red onion, peeled and very thinly sliced

a small handful of chopped mint leaves

1. Place the squid in a bowl and in another bowl, mix together the sea salt, lemon juice, ground spices, chilli powder, tomato purée, chilli, ginger and garlic. Pour this mixture over the squid. Toss to coat evenly, cover and allow to stand at room temperature for 12–15 minutes.

2. Spray a pan with Fry Light and place over a very high heat. Working in batches, lift the squid from the marinade and sear in the hot pan for 2–3 minutes. Remove and keep warm in a serving bowl while you repeat for the remaining squid.

3. Stir in the chopped coriander, red onion and chopped mint through the cooked squid, toss to mix well and eat immediately.

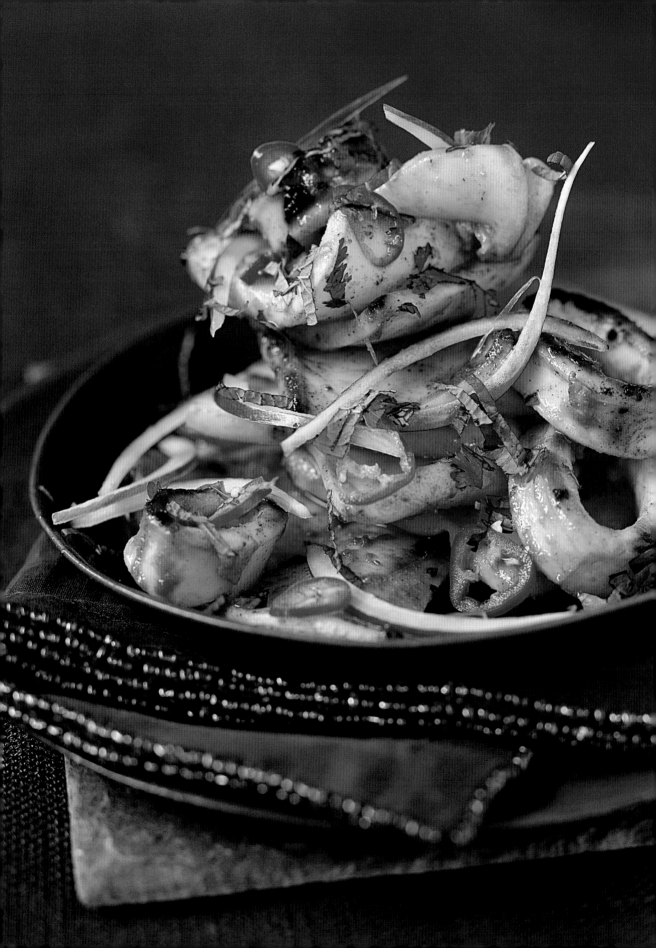

CHETTINAD PEPPER PRAWNS

VERY HOT 🌶🌶🌶🌶

This dish originated in Chettinad in southern India. It is a fiery dish of mixed peppercorns and chillies, combined with tomato, shallots and garlic. The piquancy of the green peppercorns provides an irresistible explosion of flavours and textures.

SERVES 4 ❄

Syns per serving
Original: ½

EASY
Preparation time 5 minutes
Cooking time 15 minutes

Fry Light

3 dried red chillies, roughly crushed

1 tsp crushed black peppercorns

1 tsp crushed fennel seeds or star anise

10 small shallots, peeled and finely chopped

4 garlic cloves, peeled and crushed

2 tbsp tomato purée

salt

800g/1lb 12oz raw king or tiger prawns, shelled and de-veined

2 tbsp green peppecorns (in brine) drained

1. Spray a large pan with Fry Light and place over a medium heat. Add the chilli, black peppercorns, fennel or star anise and stir-fry for 1–2 minutes.

2. Turn the heat to high and add the shallots, garlic, tomato purée and season with salt. Stir to mix well and cook for 2–3 minutes.

3. Stir in the prawns and cook for 1–2 minutes. Add 90ml/3fl oz of water, stir and cook for 3–4 minutes or until the prawns are cooked through. Remove the pan from the heat and stir in the green peppercorns just before serving with a cool cucumber salad or one of the raitas from the Accompaniments chapter (starting on page 204).

HARA JHINGA MASALA

MEDIUM ♪♪

The coastal waters of India abound with the most delicious prawns. Here they are cooked very quickly in a fresh herb and spice mixture. This is a delicious fresh masala paste for any firm white fish too.

SERVES 4 ❄
Syns per serving
Original: Free
EASY
Preparation time 10 minutes
Cooking time 5 minutes

10 tbsp finely chopped coriander leaves

6 tbsp finely chopped mint leaves

2 fresh green chillies, deseeded and finely chopped

2 tsp peeled and finely grated ginger

3 garlic cloves, peeled and crushed

Fry Light

1 tsp cumin seeds

½ tsp crushed coriander seeds

700g/1lb 8oz jumbo prawns, shelled and de-veined

salt

juice of 1 lime

1. Place the chopped coriander, mint, chilli, ginger and garlic in a small blender with a few tablespoons of water and process until smooth. (Alternatively, use a pestle and mortar.)

2. Spray a large frying pan with Fry Light and place over a high heat. Add the cumin, crushed coriander seeds and prawns and then stir-fry for 3–4 minutes or until the prawns turn pink and are cooked through.

3. Season well, squeeze over the lime juice and serve immediately.

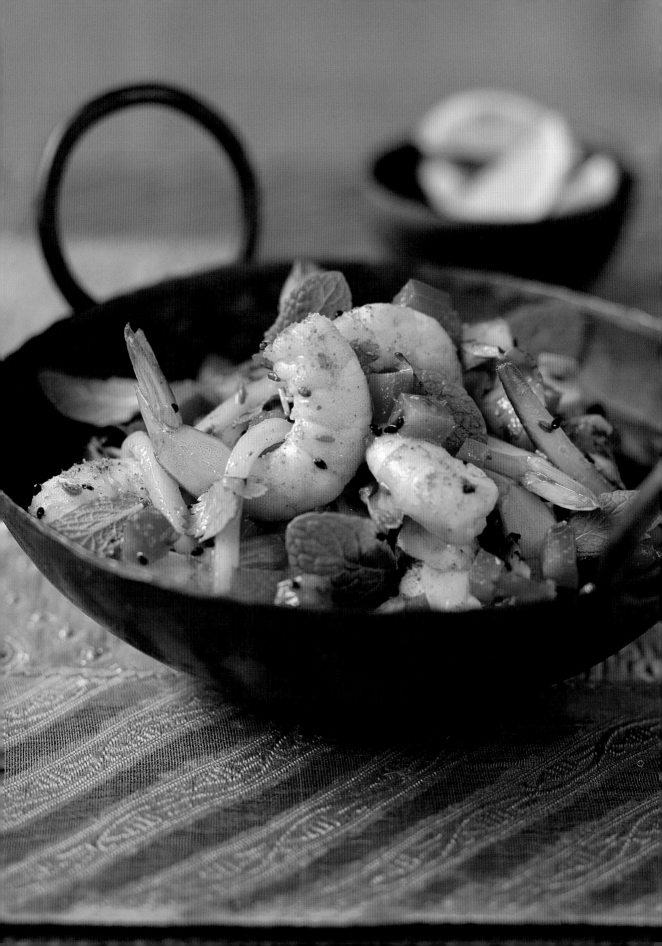

JHINGA BALTI

This quick Indian-style shrimp and vegetable stir-fry is easy to prepare and a great midweek supper stand-by. You could use any combination of vegetables.

SERVES 4 ✲
Syns per serving
Original: Free
EXTRA EASY
Preparation time 5 minutes
Cooking time 10 minutes

Fry Light

1 tsp black onion (nigella) seeds

2 tsp cumin seeds

8 fresh curry leaves

1 tsp mild curry powder

1 large cucumber, cut into matchsticks

1 red pepper, deseeded and diced

700g/1lb 8oz cooked and peeled shrimps or prawns

1 tsp crushed coriander seeds

juice of 1 lemon

salt

a small handful of mint leaves

a small handful of chopped coriander leaves

1. Spray a large pan with Fry Light and place over a medium heat. Add the black onion seeds, cumin seeds and curry leaves and stir-fry for 1–2 minutes.

2. Stir in the curry powder with the cucumber and red pepper. Stir and cook over a high heat for 4–5 minutes. Add the shrimps or prawns and the coriander seeds.

3. Stir-fry for 1–2 minutes and then squeeze over the lemon juice, season well and stir in the herbs. Remove from the heat and serve immediately.

GOAN PRAWN CURRY

HOT ///

This classic curry is part of the staple diet of the people of Goa, in southern India. The original version uses a lot of coconut milk, but here we have used reduced-fat coconut milk to great effect. Always use fresh prawns in this recipe and leave the tails on as they add to the flavour of the dish.

SERVES 4 ❄
Syns per serving
Original: 3½
EASY
Preparation time 5 minutes
Cooking time 20 minutes

1 tsp hot chilli powder

1 tbsp paprika

¼ tsp turmeric

4 garlic cloves, peeled and crushed

2 tsp peeled and finely grated ginger

2 tsp ground cumin

2 tbsp tomato purée

¼ tsp artificial sweetener

2 tsp tamarind paste

200ml/7fl oz reduced-fat coconut milk

800g/1lb 12oz tiger prawns, cleaned and shelled with the tails left on

salt and freshly ground black pepper

TO SERVE
4 tbsp finely chopped coriander leaves

1. Place the chilli powder, paprika, turmeric, garlic, ginger, cumin, tomato purée and sweetener in a saucepan and mix with 300ml/½ pint of water until smooth. Place the pan over a high heat and bring to the boil. Cover, reduce the heat and simmer gently for 8–10 minutes.

2. Stir in the tamarind paste and coconut milk and bring back to the boil. Add the prawns and cook for 6–7 minutes or until they are cooked through and have turned pink. Season well and serve immediately with the chopped coriander.

SCALLOP SAAG TAMATAR KARI

This curry is a wonderful marriage of spices, spinach and tomato with juicy, fresh scallops. If you can't find scallops, use fresh raw king prawns instead.

SERVES 4 ✷
Syns per serving
Original: Free
EASY
Preparation time 5 minutes
Cooking time 15 minutes

Fry Light

2 tsp black mustard seeds

4 garlic cloves, peeled and crushed

1 tsp peeled and finely grated ginger

1 tbsp hot curry powder

400g can chopped tomatoes

¼ tsp artificial sweetener

200g/7oz baby spinach leaves, roughly chopped

700g/1lb 8oz fresh scallops, cleaned

4 tbsp very low fat natural fromage frais

salt

1. Spray a pan with Fry Light and place over a high heat. Add the mustard seeds and as soon as they start to pop (which won't take long), add the garlic, ginger, curry powder, tomatoes, 200ml/7fl oz of water and the sweetener. Bring to the boil, reduce the heat, cover and cook for 3–4 minutes, stirring often.

2. Uncover and turn the heat to high. Add the spinach and cook for 3–4 minutes, stirring often.

3. Add the scallops and cook for 3–4 minutes until they are just cooked through. Remove from the heat, stir in the fromage frais, season well and serve immediately.

CHATNI MACCHI

This quick and impressive red mullet dish, served with a coriander, chilli and mint sauce, is perfect for last-minute entertaining. Use any fish that you want.

SERVES 4 ❋
Syns per serving
Original: Free
EASY
Preparation time 5 minutes
Cooking time 15 minutes

2 whole red mullets, scaled and cleaned

juice of 2 lemons

salt and freshly ground black pepper

2 garlic cloves, peeled and crushed

1 tsp peeled and finely grated ginger

2 tsp ground cumin

1 tsp ground coriander

1–2 fresh green chillies, deseeded and finely chopped

¼ tsp artificial sweetener

a large handful of finely chopped coriander leaves

4 tbsp finely chopped mint leaves

110g/4oz very low fat natural yogurt

TO SERVE
chopped radish
cucumber shreds
lime wedges

1. Make several diagonal cuts on each side of the fish and place on a shallow plate. Squeeze over the lemon juice and season well. Cover and set aside.

2. Make the sauce by placing all the remaining ingredients in a food processor and blending until smooth. Season and set aside.

3. Place the fish under a medium-hot grill and cook for 6–7 minutes on each side. Remove from the grill and place on a warmed serving plate. Serve immediately with the coriander, chilli and mint sauce and garnished with chopped radish and cucumber shreds, with lemon wedges to squeeze over.

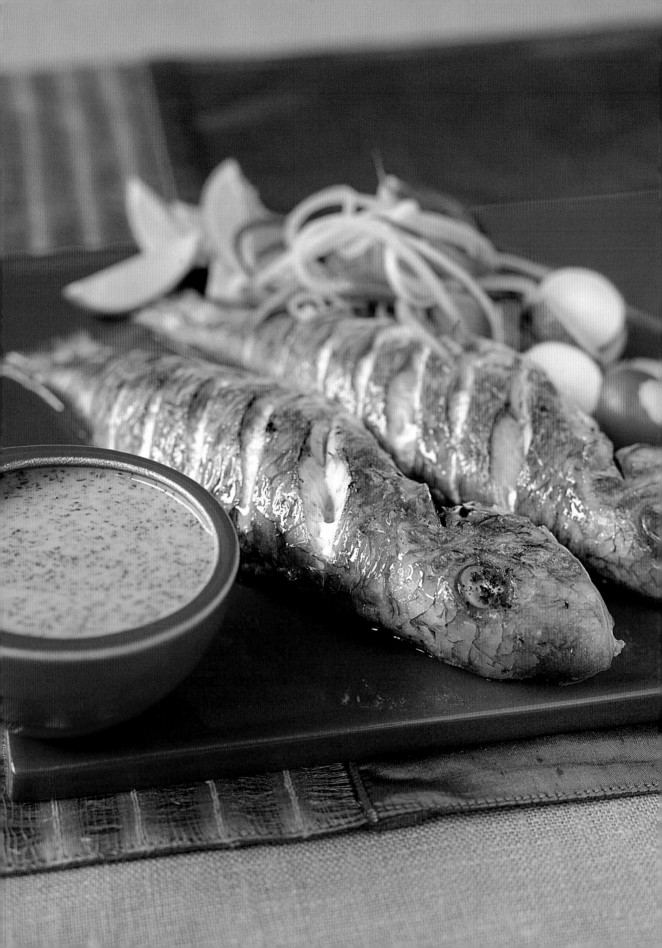

BAKED CURRIED TROUT FILLETS MILD

This dish is simplicity itself as trout fillets are lightly coated with a ready-made curry powder mixed with lime juice and yogurt and then baked until cooked through. You could use any kind of fish in place of the trout.

SERVES 4 ❄

Syns per serving
Original: Free

EASY
Preparation time 5 minutes
Cooking time 15 minutes

1 tbsp mild curry powder

juice of 1 lime

4 tbsp very low fat natural yogurt

salt

8 trout fillets, skinned

TO SERVE
lime wedges
freshly chopped mint leaves

1. Preheat the oven to 200°C/Gas 6 and line a baking tray with baking parchment.

2. In a bowl, mix together the curry powder, lime juice and yogurt. Season well with salt.

3. Spread the trout fillets in a single layer on the baking tray and spread the yogurt mixture over them evenly. Place in the preheated oven and bake for 12–15 minutes or until cooked through. Serve immediately garnished with lime wedges and mint leaves.

BENGALI BAKED FISH KEBABS MEDIUM ♪♪

This style of preparing fish and shellfish in spices and mustard seeds is typical of Bengali cuisine in eastern India. Usually they use a fresh water fish called hilsa, but here we have used halibut. Cod or any other firm, white-fleshed fish will make a good alternative.

SERVES 4 ❄

Syns per serving
Original: 1½

EASY
Preparation time 10 minutes
(plus standing)
Cooking time 12 minutes

2 tsp black mustard seeds

2 tsp yellow mustard seeds

2 tbsp peeled and very finely chopped onion

1 fresh green chilli, deseeded and finely chopped

1 fresh red chilli, deseeded and finely chopped

½ tsp turmeric

2 tsp sea salt

¼ tsp mild or medium chilli powder

juice of 2 lemons

1 tbsp mustard oil

800g/1lb 12oz thick halibut fillets, skinned and cut into bite-sized pieces

Fry Light

1. Combine the mustard seeds, onion, chillies, turmeric, salt, chilli powder, lemon juice and mustard oil and 1–2 tablespoons of water and, using a pestle and mortar, mix to a coarse, rough paste.

2. Preheat the oven to 200°C/Gas 6. Place the fish in a bowl and add the mustard mixture to it. Using your fingers, toss to mix and coat evenly, cover and let stand for 10–15 minutes to allow the flavours to develop.

3. Thread the fish onto 12 wooden skewers and place on a baking tray lined with baking parchment. Spray lightly with Fry Light and bake for 10–12 minutes or until the fish is just cooked through and opaque. Remove from the oven and serve immediately.

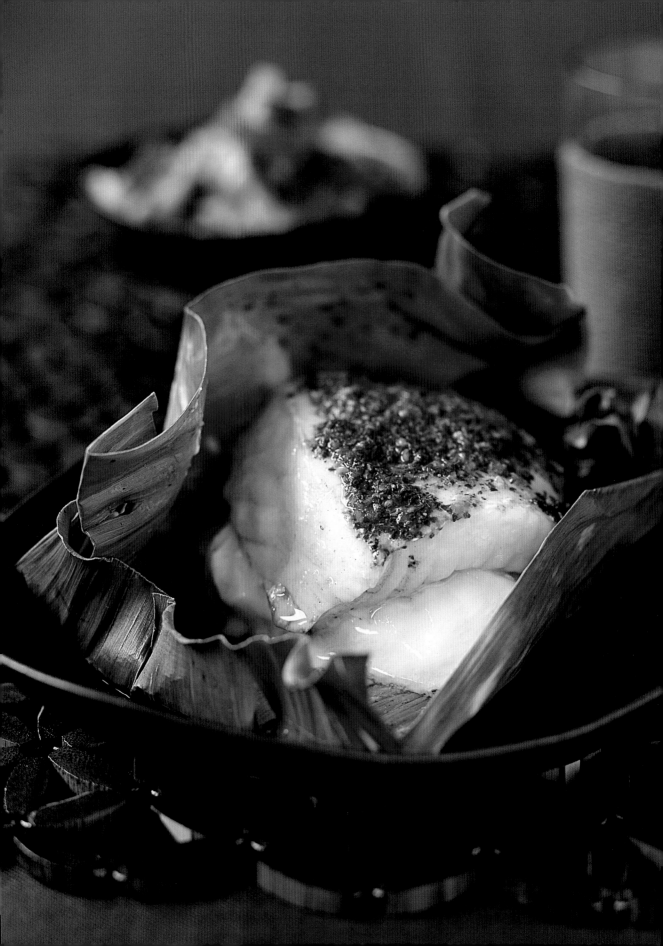

KERALA-STYLE FISH STEAMED IN BANANA LEAVES

MEDIUM

This dish is a typical speciality from Kerala (a coastal state that has seafood and banana plantations in abundance). Steaming the fish allows you to enjoy its full flavour and the banana leaves add a special essence to the fish dish. If you can't find banana leaves, baking parchment is a good alternative.

SERVES 4
Syns per serving
Original: Free
WORTH THE EFFORT
Preparation time 10 minutes
Cooking time 10 minutes

4 thick white fish fillets (halibut, cod or monkfish), skinless

4 large pieces of banana leaf or baking parchment

110g/4oz coriander leaves, chopped

5 tbsp chopped mint leaves

1 onion, peeled and chopped

1 tsp peeled and finely grated ginger

2 fresh green chillies, deseeded and finely chopped

finely grated zest and juice of 1 large lime

salt

1. Pat the fish dry and place on a plate. Heat the banana leaf over an open flame (if using) until it turns bright green and becomes supple. Remove and set aside.

2. Put the coriander, mint, onion, ginger, chilli, lime zest and juice in a food processor. Season well, add a little water and blend until fairly smooth. Spread this mixture over the fish, cover and allow to marinate for 10–12 minutes.

3. Place a large steamer over a pan of simmering water. Lay the fish on the banana leaf (or baking parchment) with the marinade and wrap up to make a parcel enclosing the fish. Secure with small skewers and place the parcel in the steamer, cover and cook for 10–12 minutes or until the fish is opaque and cooked through.

4. To serve, carefully remove the parcel from the steamer and unwrap at the table so that everyone can savour the aroma. This tastes great served with Kachumber (see page 212)

TIP You can bake the fish instead of steaming it if you prefer. Place the fish parcel on a non-stick baking sheet and bake at 190°C/Gas 5 for 10–15 minutes.

TALI MACCHI

In this simple but satisfying fish recipe, cod steaks or fillets are seasoned with spices and simply cooked on a hot griddle or pan. You could use any fish of your choice here, bearing in mind that firm, white-fleshed fish works best.

SERVES 4 ❄
Syns per serving
Original: 1
EASY
Preparation time 5 minutes
(plus standing)
Cooking time 10 minutes

4 cod steaks or thick fillets, skinless
2 tsp sea salt
1 tsp crushed black peppercorns
½ tsp turmeric
¼ tsp mild chilli powder
1 tsp roughly crushed cumin seeds
1 tsp roughly crushed coriander seeds
½ tsp garam masala
1 tbsp plain flour
Fry Light

TO SERVE
lime wedges
freshly chopped mint leaves

1. Place the fish in a single layer on a large plate. Mix together the salt, peppercorns, turmeric, chilli powder, cumin seeds, coriander seeds and garam masala and dust both sides of the fish with this mixture.

2. Rub the spices into the fish and then lightly dust with the flour. Cover and leave to rest for 10–15 minutes at room temperature.

3. Spray a large pan with Fry Light and place over a high heat. Add the fish and cook for 4–5 minutes on each side until cooked through. Serve immediately with lime wedges and mint leaves.

TAMARIND AND SALMON CURRY

MEDIUM ♪♪

Tamarind comes from the pod of a large tree and usually you can buy it in blocks from Asian greengrocers. It adds a very tangy flavour to this curry and enhances the flavours of the spices used. You can now buy ready-bottled tamarind paste in all major supermarkets but if you cannot get hold of it, use the juice of a lime or lemon instead.

SERVES 4 ❋

Syns per serving
Original: 3½

EASY
Preparation time 10 minutes
Cooking time 10 minutes

Fry Light

2 garlic cloves, peeled and thinly sliced

2 tsp cumin seeds

1 tsp black mustard seeds

1 tsp crushed coriander seeds

12–15 fresh curry leaves

750g/1lb 10oz salmon fillet, skinned and cut into bite-sized pieces

2 tbsp tomato purée

¼ tsp artificial sweetener

1 tsp garam masala

1 tsp ground cumin

8 tbsp finely chopped coriander leaves

2 fresh red chillies, deseeded and finely sliced

2 tsp tamarind paste

200ml/7fl oz reduced-fat coconut milk

salt

1. Spray a large saucepan with Fry Light and place over a medium heat. Add the garlic, cumin, mustard seeds, coriander seeds and curry leaves and stir-fry for 1–2 minutes.

2. Add the salmon to the pan. Mix the remaining ingredients (except the salt) and pour into the pan. Turn the heat to medium-low. Cover and allow the mixture to simmer and cook for 6–8 minutes or until the fish is cooked through.

3. Remove the pan from the heat, season the food well with salt and serve immediately.

SONF MACCHI

Salmon steaks, cooked in a lightly spiced fennel-flavoured sauce, makes for a healthy lunch when served with a salad. You can use any other thick fish fillet or steak if desired. The Indian word for fennel is sonf.

SERVES 4 ❀
Syns per serving
Original: Free

EASY
Preparation time 5 minutes
Cooking time 20 minutes

Fry Light

10 fresh curry leaves

1 red onion, peeled and finely chopped

2 tsp peeled and finely grated garlic

1 tsp peeled and finely grated ginger

1 tbsp fennel seeds

1 tbsp mild curry powder

5 large ripe tomatoes, deseeded and chopped

4 thick salmon steaks or fillets, skinless

salt

TO SERVE
freshly chopped coriander leaves
red onion slices

1. Spray a large pan with Fry Light and place over a high heat. Add the curry leaves and onion and stir-fry for 4–5 minutes.

2. Turn the heat to medium-low and add the garlic, ginger, fennel seeds and curry powder. Stir-fry for 2–3 minutes.

3. Turn the heat to high and add the tomatoes and stir-fry for 3–4 minutes. Place the salmon steaks in the pan in a single layer, spoon over some of the sauce, season well, simmer and cook gently for 7–8 minutes or until cooked through. Remove from the heat and serve immediately garnished with coriander leaves and red onion slices.

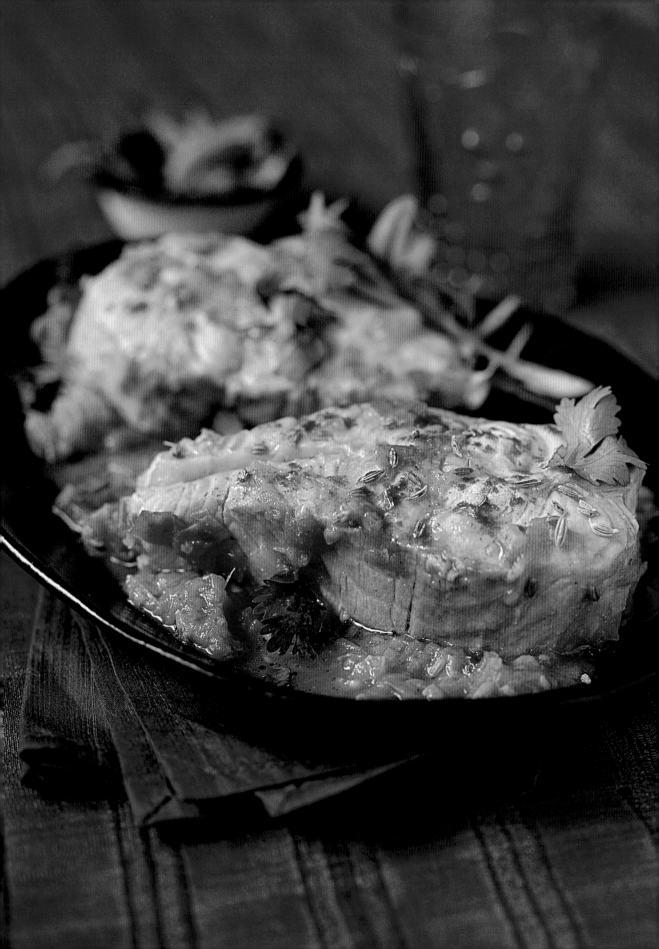

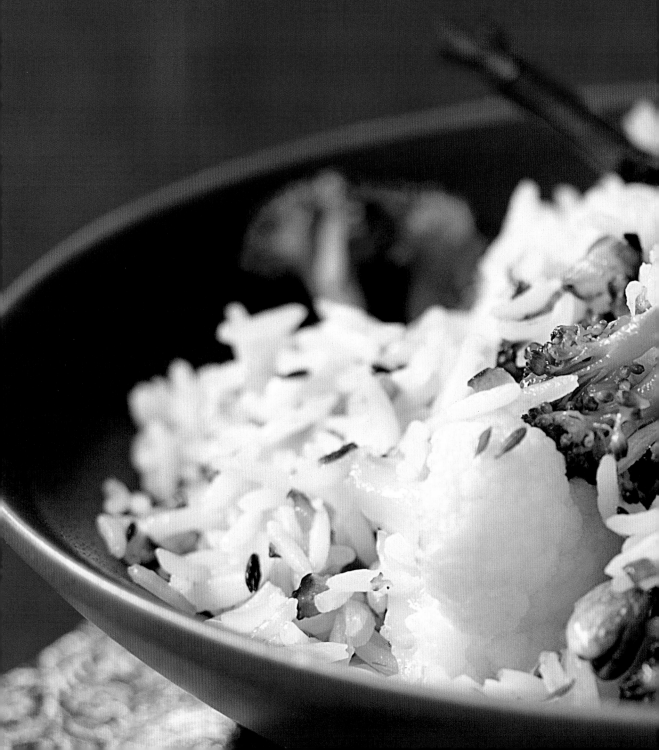

RICE, LENTILS AND PULSES

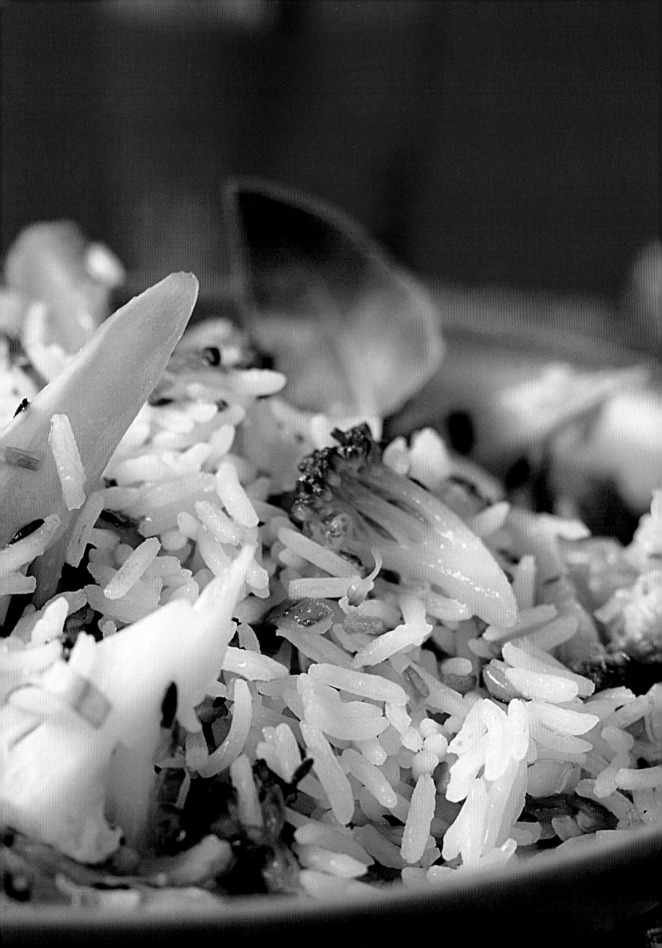

TOMATO AND MUSHROOM RICE

MILD ✎

This delicious dish is great to eat on its own or can be served with vegetables or a salad. You could use any type of fresh mushrooms that you wish.

SERVES 4 ⓥ ❄
Syns per serving
Green: ½

EASY
Preparation time 5 minutes (plus soaking)
Cooking time 20 minutes (plus standing)

225g/8oz basmati rice
Fry Light
2 tsp cumin seeds
3 tbsp peeled and finely chopped onion
110g/4oz fresh mushrooms, roughly sliced or chopped
3 tbsp tomato purée
¼ tsp crushed cardamom seeds
1 tsp ground cinnamon
4–5 black peppercorns
1 bay leaf
salt

1. Wash the rice in cold water, place in a bowl and cover with more cold water. Allow the rice to soak for 30 minutes, then drain and set aside.

2. Spray a large pan with Fry Light and place over a medium heat. Add the cumin seeds and stir-fry for 1 minute before adding the onion. Stir and cook for 2–3 minutes, turn the heat to high and add the mushrooms. Stir for 1–2 minutes and then add the rice, 450ml/16fl oz of water, the tomato purée, cardamom seeds, cinnamon, black peppercorns and bay leaf.

3. Season well and bring to the boil. Cover tightly, reduce the heat to very low and cook for 12–15 minutes, undisturbed. Remove from the heat and allow to stand for 10 minutes before serving.

TIP To make a delicious carrot rice, use coarsely grated carrots instead of the mushrooms.

SPICY FISH PILAU

Spiced fish and fragrant basmati rice are baked together to make this traditional one-pot dish, which makes for stress-free, yet elegant, entertaining.

SERVES 4 ❋
Syns per serving
Green: Free
(add 6 Syns if not using cod as a
Healthy Extra)

WORTH THE EFFORT
Preparation time 10 minutes
Cooking time 40 minutes

4 x 175g/6oz cod fillets, skinless,
cut into bite-sized pieces

2 tbsp lemon juice

4 spring onions, trimmed and
finely chopped

1 fresh red chilli, deseeded and
thinly sliced

1 tsp ground fennel seeds

½ tsp mild or medium chilli
powder

2 tsp ground cumin

4 garlic cloves, peeled and
crushed

1 tsp peeled and finely grated
ginger

½ tsp turmeric

salt and freshly ground black
pepper

350g/12oz basmati rice

2 bay leaves

1 cinnamon stick

TO SERVE
4 tbsp chopped fresh coriander
leaves

1. Place the cod in a bowl. Mix together the lemon juice, spring onions, chilli, fennel seeds, chilli powder, cumin, garlic, ginger, turmeric and seasoning and pour over the fish. Toss to mix well.

2. Heat the oven to 150°C/Gas 2. Rinse and drain the rice. Bring 600ml/1 pint of water to the boil in a saucepan and add the bay leaves and cinnamon and season well with salt. Add the rice and return to the boil for 3 minutes or until the water has been absorbed. Take the pan off the heat and leave it uncovered for 5 minutes.

3. Place a few pieces of the fish and some marinade in a casserole dish. Cover with a layer of rice and continue layering with the fish and rice, finishing with the rice.

4. Cover the mixture with baking parchment and then with foil and cover tightly with the casserole lid. Bake in the preheated oven for 20–25 minutes. Remove from the oven and serve garnished with the chopped coriander.

TIP You can replace the fennel seeds, chilli powder and ground cumin with 2 tbsp medium curry powder if liked.

JATPATTA PHOOL GOBI CHAWAL

MILD ✒

This is a quick Indian-style rice and vegetable stir-fry dish that uses cooked leftover vegetables and rice flavoured with aromatic spices. We've used cauliflower and broccoli in this recipe but feel free to use any leftover vegetables that you have to hand.

SERVES 4 Ⓥ ❋
Syns per serving
Green: Free

EXTRA EASY
Preparation time 5 minutes
Cooking time 15 minutes

Fry Light

2 tbsp peeled and finely chopped red onion

1 cinnamon stick

1 bay leaf

3 green cardamom pods, crushed

1 tsp cumin seeds

2 cloves

400g/14oz boiled cauliflower and broccoli florets

500g/1lb 2oz boiled brown or white basmati rice

salt and freshly ground black pepper

1. Spray a large wok with Fry Light and place over a high heat. Add the onion, cinnamon stick, bay leaf, cardamom pods, cumin seeds and cloves and stir-fry for 3–4 minutes.

2. Add the cauliflower and broccoli florets to the wok and stir-fry for 1–2 minutes.

3. Add the cooked rice and stir-fry over a high heat for 4–5 minutes or until piping hot. Season and serve immediately.

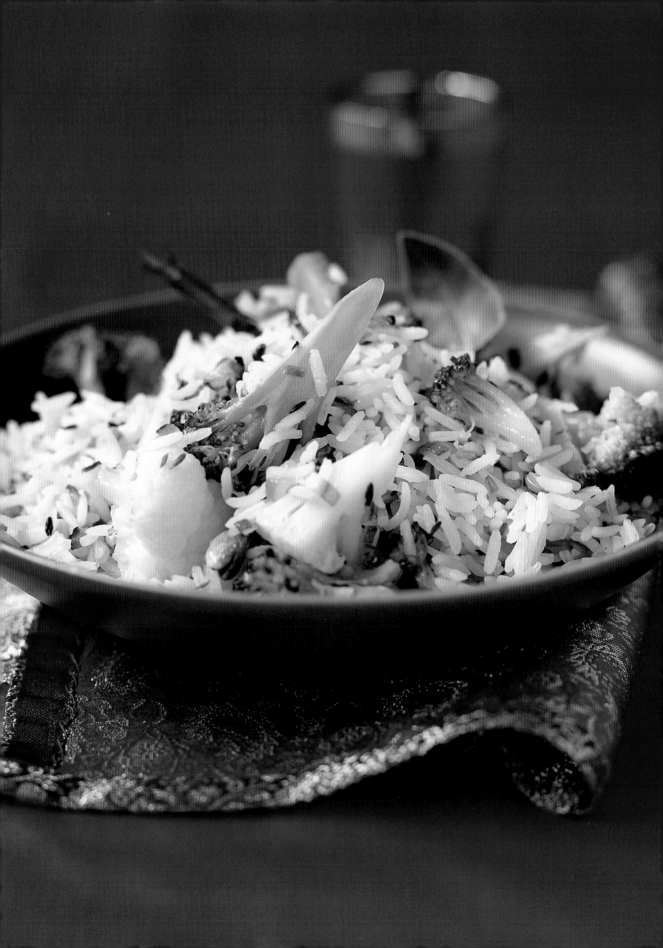

LEMON AND TURMERIC RICE

MEDIUM 🌶🌶

A wonderfully flavoured and coloured rice that will make an ideal partner for a range of spicy dishes.

SERVES 4 Ⓥ ❄

Syns per serving
Green: Free

EASY
Preparation time 5 minutes
(plus soaking)
Cooking time 20 minutes
(plus standing)

225g/8oz basmati rice

Fry Light

2 tsp black mustard seeds

2 dried red chillies, roughly crumbled

1 tsp turmeric

finely grated zest and juice of 1 lemon

3 tbsp finely chopped coriander leaves

salt

1. Rinse the rice and place in a bowl and cover with cold water. Leave to soak for 20–30 minutes, then drain in a sieve.

2. Spray a large saucepan with Fry Light and when hot, add the mustard seeds. As soon as they start to 'pop' add the chilli and stir-fry for 30–40 seconds.

3. Add the rice and turmeric and stir-fry for 2–3 minutes. Add the lemon zest and juice and coriander leaves. Season well with salt and pour over 450ml/16fl oz of boiling hot water. Bring to the boil, cover tightly, reduce the heat to very low and cook, undisturbed, for 10 minutes. Fluff up the grains with a fork before serving.

PEA PILAU

A popular rice speciality from India, this dish can be made with either fresh or frozen peas. Lightly spiced, this serves as a great accompaniment to any vegetable or lentil dish or can be eaten on its own with a salad.

SERVES 4 Ⓥ ❄

Syns per serving
Green: Free

EASY
Preparation time 5 minutes
Cooking time 25 minutes
(plus standing)

Fry Light

1 onion, peeled, halved and very thinly sliced

4–5 cloves

2 dried bay leaves

6–8 cardamom pods, lightly crushed

5cm/2in stick of cinnamon

1 tbsp cumin seeds

175g/6oz fresh or frozen garden peas

400g/14oz basmati rice

salt

1. Spray a large pan with Fry Light and place over a medium heat. Add the onion and stir-fry for 4–5 minutes or until soft and lightly browned.

2. Add the cloves, bay leaves, cardamom pods, cinnamon and cumin seeds and stir-fry for 2–3 minutes. Add the peas and rice and stir-fry for another 1–2 minutes.

3. Pour in 750ml/26fl oz of boiling water, season well and bring to the boil. Cover tightly, reduce the heat to very low and cook, undisturbed, for 12–15 minutes. Remove from the heat and allow to stand, again undisturbed, for 10–12 minutes.

4. To serve, uncover and fluff up the grains of rice with a fork and serve immediately.

TIP Canned chickpeas make a delicious alternative to the garden peas.

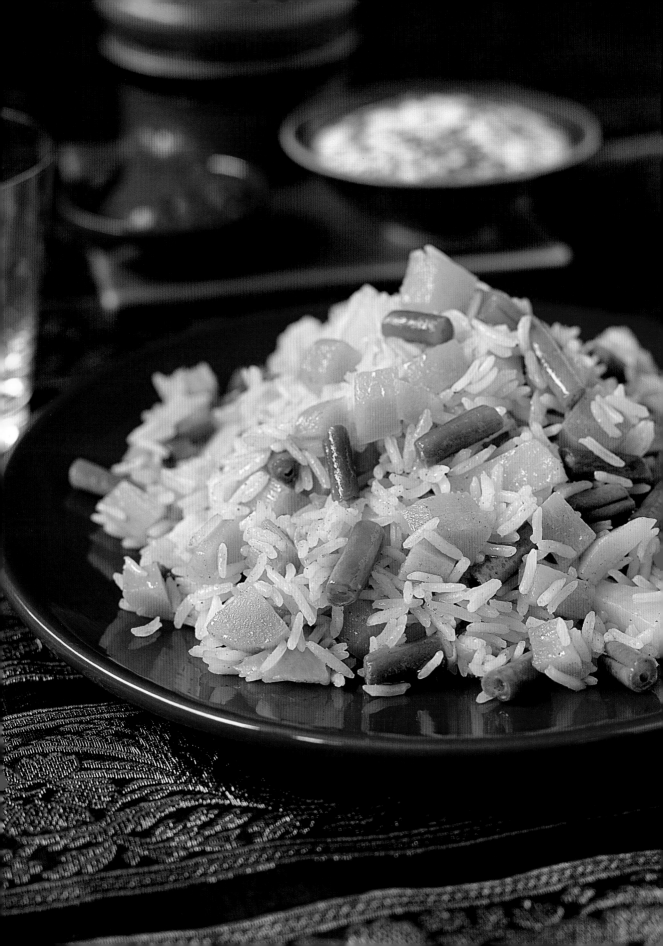

MIXED VEGETABLE BIRYANI

MILD ✏

A mixture of vegetables cooked with fragrant basmati rice makes this one-pot classic recipe a perfect entertaining dish. Use any combination of vegetables that you like.

SERVES 4 Ⓥ ❄
Syns per serving
Green: Free
EASY
Preparation time 5 minutes
Cooking time 30 minutes

Fry Light

1 onion, peeled and finely chopped

1 tsp peeled and finely grated ginger

2 garlic cloves, peeled and crushed

½ tsp turmeric

1 tsp mild chilli powder

1 tsp ground cumin

1 tsp ground coriander

1 tsp crushed cardamom seeds

1 tsp ground cinnamon

2 cloves

1 carrot, peeled and finely chopped

110g/4oz fine green beans, trimmed and chopped

1 potato, peeled and finely chopped

4 tbsp very low fat natural yogurt

110g/4oz basmati rice

salt

1. Spray a pan with Fry Light and place over a medium heat. Add the onion and stir-fry for 5–6 minutes until softened and lightly browned.

2. Add the ginger, garlic, turmeric, chilli powder, cumin, coriander, cardamom seeds, cinnamon and cloves and stir-fry for 2–3 minutes. Add the vegetables and yogurt and stir and cook gently for 2–3 minutes. Add the rice and stir-fry for a further 2–3 minutes. Season well.

3. Pour 200ml/7fl oz of boiling water over the vegetables and rice and bring to the boil. Cover tightly and reduce the heat to very low. Cook undisturbed for 12–15 minutes and then remove from the heat and allow to stand, again undisturbed, for 10 minutes.

4. To serve, uncover and fluff up the grains of rice with a fork. Eat the biryani immediately.

KITCHEREE

Red split lentils, which require no pre-soaking, are cooked with rice, spices and potatoes to produce a delicious Indian-style risotto, which is the ultimate in comfort food.

SERVES 4 ⓥ ❋
Syns per serving
Green: Free

EASY
Preparation time 5 minutes
Cooking time 20 minutes
(plus standing)

Fry Light

5–6 cloves

2 tsp cumin seeds

1 cinnamon stick

½ tsp cardamom seeds

¼ tsp turmeric

2 tsp sea salt

150g/5oz red split lentils
(masoor dal), washed and
drained

110g/4oz basmati rice

1 large potato, peeled and finely
diced

1 small onion, peeled, halved
and thinly sliced

1. Spray a large pan with Fry Light and place over a medium heat. Add the cloves, cumin seeds, cinnamon stick and cardamom seeds and stir-fry for 2–3 minutes.

2. Add the turmeric, salt, lentils, rice, potato and onion and stir-fry for 2–3 minutes.

3. Pour over 300ml/½ pint of water and bring to the boil. Cover tightly, turn the heat to low and cook undisturbed for 12–15 minutes. Remove from the heat and allow to stand, again undisturbed, for 10 minutes. To serve, fluff up the rice grains with a fork and serve immediately.

SAAMBHAR

This soup-like vegetable curry is tangy and spicy and comes from southern India. Saambhar powder is widely available in all good Indian greengrocers, but if you are unable to find it, use a mild curry powder instead.

SERVES 4 Ⓥ ❄
Syns per serving
Green: Free
WORTH THE EFFORT
Preparation time 5 minutes
Cooking time 45 minutes

110g/4oz yellow split lentils, washed and drained

½ tsp turmeric

1 aubergine, cut into bite-sized pieces

1 potato, peeled and cut into bite-sized pieces

1 carrot, peeled and cut into bite-sized pieces

Fry Light

1 small onion, peeled and chopped

2 garlic cloves, peeled and crushed

10 tsp black mustard seeds

10 fresh curry leaves

½ tsp crushed black peppercorns

2 small dried red chillies

1 tbsp saambhar powder or mild curry powder

1 tomato, cut into wedges

1 tsp tamarind paste

salt

1. Place the lentils, turmeric and 800ml/28fl oz of water in a saucepan and bring to the boil. Cover and cook on a gentle heat for 40–45 minutes, adding the aubergine, potato and carrot halfway through the cooking time.

2. While the lentils are cooking, spray a frying pan with Fry Light and place over a medium heat. Add the onion, stir and cook for 6–8 minutes or until softened. Add the garlic, mustard seeds, curry leaves, peppercorns, red chillies, saambhar or curry powder and cook for 1–2 minutes. Stir in the tomato and cook for 3–4 minutes.

3. Add this mixture to the lentils with the tamarind, season well and stir to combine. Bring back to the boil and cook for 2–3 minutes until piping hot. Serve ladled into warm bowls and eat immediately.

SPINACH DHAL

MEDIUM ♪♪

Yellow split lentils (moong dal) are used in this hearty lentil curry, but you could always substitute them with red split lentils if liked.

SERVES 4 Ⓥ ❄
Syns per serving
Green: Free

WORTH THE EFFORT
Preparation time 5 minutes
Cooking time 35 minutes

250g/9oz yellow split lentils, washed and drained

200g/7oz baby spinach leaves, roughly chopped

Fry Light

4 shallots, peeled and very finely chopped

1 tsp peeled and finely chopped ginger

2 fresh red chillies, deseeded and finely sliced

8–10 fresh curry leaves

½ tsp turmeric

4 plum tomatoes, roughly chopped

salt

1. Place the lentils in a saucepan with 700ml/24fl oz of hot water and bring to the boil, skimming off any scum that comes to the surface. Reduce the heat to medium-low and cook for 20–25 minutes, stirring often to ensure that the thickened lentils do not stick to the bottom of the pan.

2. Add the spinach, stir, cover and cook gently for 5–6 minutes.

3. Meanwhile, spray a frying pan with Fry Light and place over a medium heat. Add the shallots and stir-fry for 4–5 minutes and then add the ginger, chilli and curry leaves. Stir-fry for 2–3 minutes, add the turmeric and stir. Scrape the contents of the frying pan into the lentils, add the tomatoes and cook on a medium heat for 4–5 minutes. Season well and serve immediately.

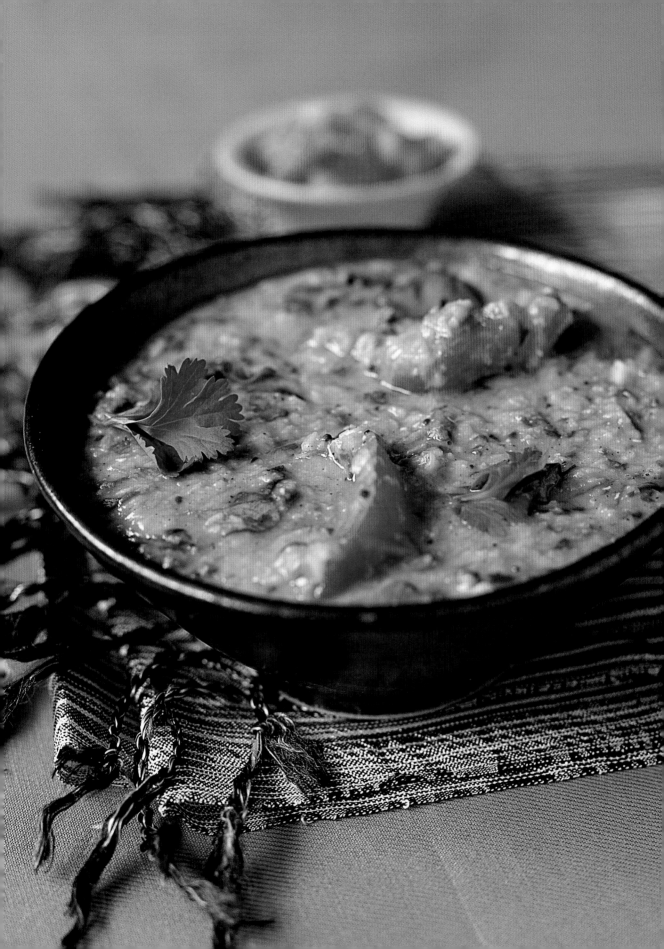

COURGETTE AND
LENTIL CURRY

MEDIUM 🌶🌶

The fresh flavour of the courgettes marries well with the nutty flavour of the lentils used in this healthy dish. In India, various different kinds of squash are used instead of the courgettes.

SERVES 4 Ⓥ ❄

Syns per serving
Green: Free

EASY
Preparation time 5 minutes
Cooking time 40 minutes

Fry Light

6 green cardamom pods, lightly crushed

2 tsp cumin seeds

3 cloves

1 red onion, peeled and finely diced

4 garlic cloves, peeled and crushed

1 tsp peeled and finely grated ginger

2 fresh red chillies, deseeded and sliced

225g/8oz yellow split lentils, washed and drained

1 tsp turmeric

2 tsp ground cumin

2 courgettes, cut into bite-sized pieces

2 tomatoes, roughly chopped

a large handful of chopped coriander leaves

salt

1. Spray a large saucepan with Fry Light and place over a medium heat. Add the cardamom pods, cumin seeds and cloves and stir-fry for 30–40 seconds. Then add the onion, garlic, ginger, chillies and stir-fry for a further 4–5 minutes.

2. Add the lentils, turmeric and ground cumin and stir-fry for 3–4 minutes. Pour over 600ml/1 pint of hot water, cover and reduce the heat to low. Cook for 20–25 minutes, stirring occasionally.

3. Add the courgettes, stir and cook for 4–5 minutes.

4. Remove the saucepan from the heat, stir in the tomatoes and chopped coriander, season well and serve immediately.

TARKA DHAL

MEDIUM ⸝⸝

Tarka is the Indian process of tempering the spices in oil to flavour dishes like lentils. Here we temper the spices in Fry Light to create a simple, every-day staple of the Indian diet.

SERVES 4 Ⓥ ❄
Syns per serving
Green: Free

WORTH THE EFFORT
Preparation time 5 minutes
Cooking time 45 minutes

350g/12oz red split lentils, washed and drained

½ tsp turmeric

1 tsp peeled and finely grated ginger

Fry Light

1 tsp cumin seeds

1 tsp black mustard seeds

1–2 dried red chillies

2 garlic cloves, peeled and finely chopped

salt

6 tbsp chopped coriander leaves

1. Place the lentils in a large saucepan with the turmeric, ginger and 1.25 litres/2 pints of water. Stir and bring to a simmer but don't let it come to the boil. Skim off any scum that comes to the surface. Continue to simmer gently for 35–40 minutes, stirring a few times during cooking. Remove from the heat and set aside.

2. Spray a small frying pan with Fry Light and place on a medium-high heat. Add the cumin and mustard seeds and as soon as they start to 'pop', add the red chillies and garlic. Stir and cook for 1–2 minutes and then add to the lentil mixture.

3. Return to the heat, season well and bring to the boil. Remove from the heat, stir in the coriander and serve immediately.

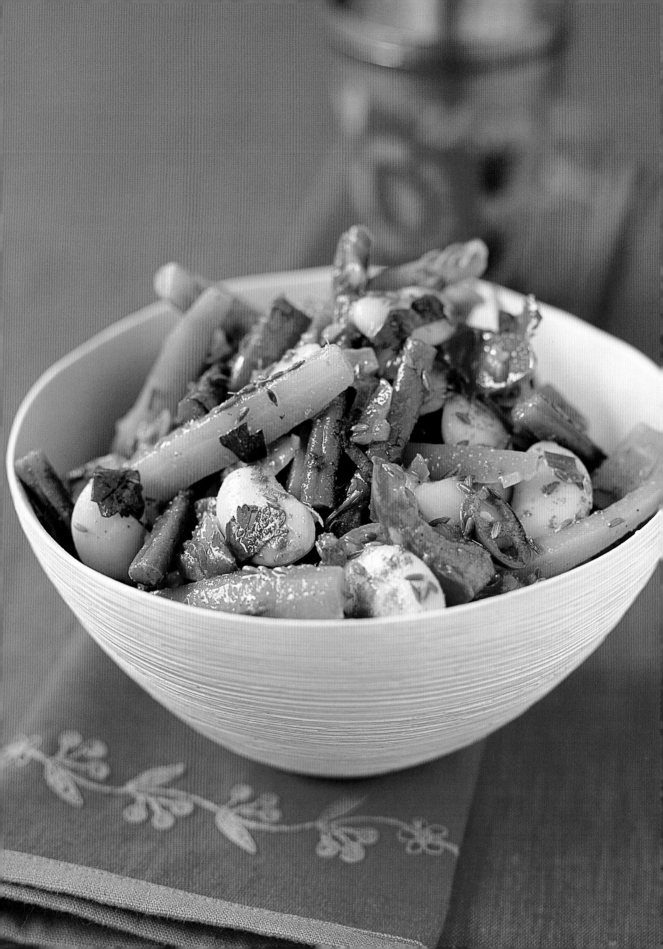

MIXED BEAN AND CARROT SABZI

MILD

This colourful and quick stir-fry is packed with protein and fibre. Butter beans, fresh green beans and carrots are swiftly cooked with spices and herbs. For this dish, which uses cooked carrots and green beans, they are cooked in boiling water for 6–7 minutes or until just tender, drained and set aside to use later. Sabzi is one of the Indian terms for vegetables.

SERVES 4 Ⓥ ❄
Syns per serving
Green: Free

EXTRA EASY
Preparation time 15 minutes
Cooking time 15 minutes

Fry Light

1 tsp cumin seeds

1 small onion, peeled and finely chopped

2 garlic cloves, peeled and finely chopped

1 tsp peeled and finely grated ginger

1 fresh green chilli, deseeded and sliced

1 fresh tomato, roughly chopped

2 tsp mild curry powder

200g/7oz carrots, cut into thick batons, boiled and drained

200g/7oz green beans, trimmed, halved, boiled and drained

200g can butter beans, rinsed and drained

salt

4 tbsp finely chopped coriander leaves

1. Spray a large frying pan with Fry Light and place over a medium heat. Add the cumin seeds, onion, garlic, ginger and chilli and stir-fry for 4–5 minutes.

2. Turn the heat to high and add the tomato, curry powder and 150ml/5fl oz of water. Stir and cook for 2–3 minutes.

3. Add the carrots, green beans and butter beans and cook for a further 3–4 minutes. Remove from the heat, season well and stir in the chopped coriander just before serving.

BLACK-EYED BEAN CURRY

Canned black-eyed beans are extremely handy to use in this quick curry, which can be prepared in a hurry.

SERVES 4 Ⓥ ❋
Syns per serving
Green: Free
EXTRA EASY
Preparation time 5 minutes
Cooking time 20 minutes

Fry Light

1 tsp black mustard seeds

1 tsp cumin seeds

1 tsp peeled and finely grated ginger

1 tbsp medium curry powder

1 small red pepper, deseeded and finely diced

200g can chopped tomatoes

¼ tsp artificial sweetener

1 tsp tamarind paste

400g can black-eyed beans, rinsed and drained

2 tbsp trimmed and chopped spring onions

salt

1. Spray a pan with Fry Light and place over a medium heat. Add the mustard and cumin seeds and stir-fry for 1–2 minutes. Add the ginger, curry powder and red pepper and stir-fry for another 1–2 minutes.

2. Add the tomatoes, sweetener and tamarind paste. Stir and cook for 2–3 minutes.

3. Add the beans along with 175ml/6fl oz of water, stir well, cover and cook for 10 minutes. Stir in the spring onions, season well, remove from the heat and serve hot.

RAJMA

MEDIUM

Another traditional Indian bean dish, here red kidney beans are cooked with herbs and spices.

SERVES 4 Ⓥ ❄

Syns per serving
Green: Free

EASY
Preparation time 5 minutes
Cooking time 15 minutes

1 small onion, peeled and finely grated

1 tsp peeled and finely grated ginger

4 garlic cloves, peeled and crushed

Fry Light

2 tsp ground cumin

2 tsp ground coriander

1 tsp mild or medium chilli powder

1 tbsp tomato purée

400g can red kidney beans, rinsed and drained

4 tbsp chopped coriander leaves

salt

4 tbsp very low fat natural fromage frais

1. Mix together the onion, ginger and garlic. Spray a pan with Fry Light and place over a medium heat. Add the onion mixture and stir-fry for 4–5 minutes. Reduce the heat to low and add the ground cumin and coriander, chilli powder and tomato purée. Stir-fry for another 1–2 minutes.

2. Add the beans and increase the heat to high. Add 200ml/7fl oz of water and cook, stirring often, for 4–5 minutes.

3. Remove from the heat and stir in the chopped coriander. Season well and just before serving, stir in the fromage frais.

CHANA MASALA

MEDIUM 🌶🌶

This tasty and healthy dish of spiced chickpeas makes a great meal when served on its own or with a salad or rice dish. It originates in the northern Indian state of Punjab.

SERVES 4 Ⓥ ❄
Syns per serving
Green: Free
EASY
Preparation time 5 minutes
Cooking time 25 minutes

Fry Light

1 cinnamon stick

3cm/1¼in piece of ginger, peeled and cut into thin shreds

6 garlic cloves, peeled and crushed

1 fresh green chilli, deseeded and thinly sliced

1 small onion, peeled and finely chopped

1 tbsp medium curry powder

110g/4oz passata

1 large potato, peeled and cut into cubes

400g can chickpeas, drained and rinsed

a squeeze of lemon juice

¼ tsp garam masala

salt

2 tbsp chopped mint leaves

2 tbsp chopped coriander leaves

1. Spray a large frying pan with Fry Light and place over a medium heat. Add the cinnamon, ginger, garlic and most of the chilli and stir-fry for 1 minute. Add the onion and cook for 6–7 minutes or until softened.

2. Add the curry powder and stir-fry for 1 minute and then add the passata, 150ml/5fl oz of hot water and the potatoes. Stir and bring to the boil, cover and reduce the heat to low. Cook gently for 10–12 minutes and then add the chickpeas and cook for 5 minutes or until the potatoes are tender.

3. Remove from the heat, sprinkle over the lemon juice and garam masala, season well and stir in the chopped herbs. Serve garnished with the remaining chilli.

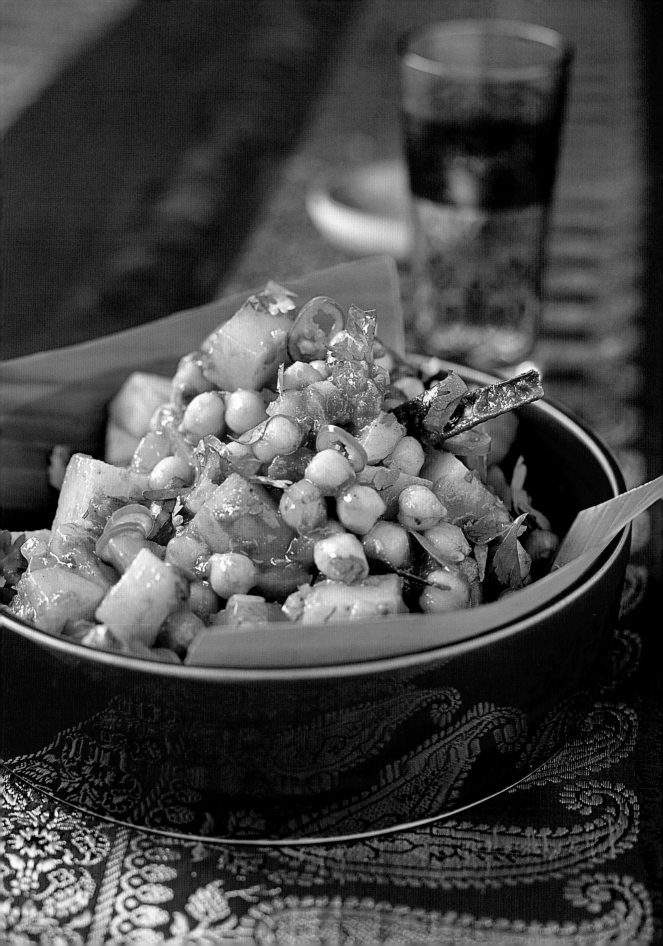

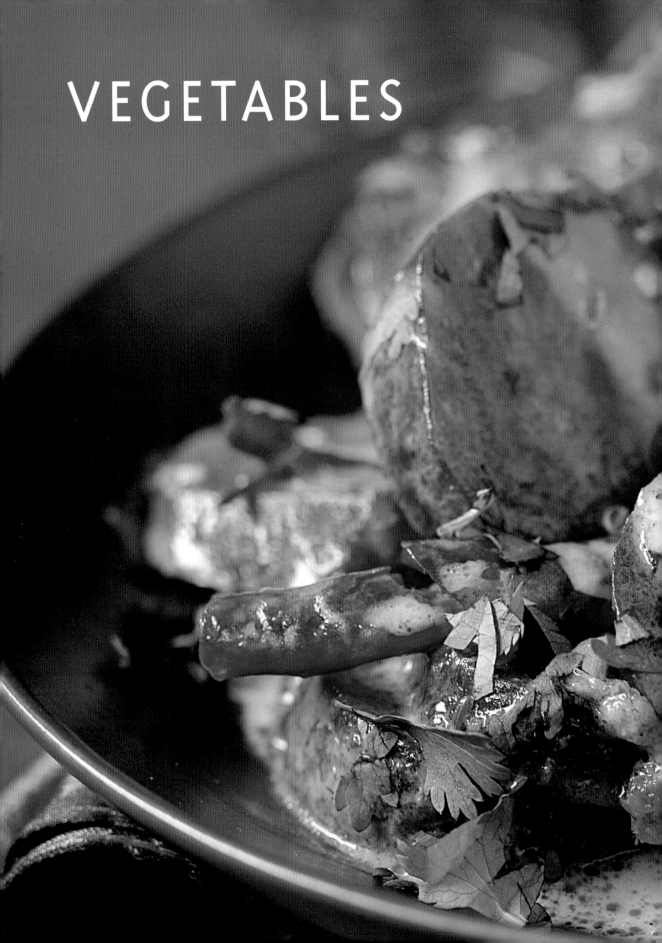

VEGETABLES

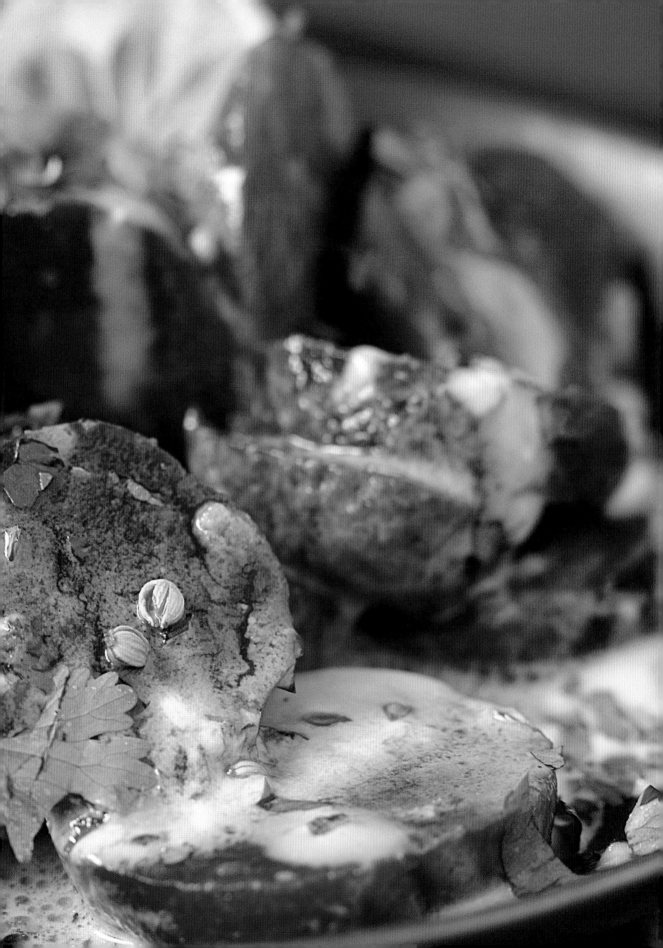

ACHARI BAINGAN

This moist and delicious dish of spiced aubergines will convert anybody who is not sure of the magnificent vegetable. In this recipe, we have used baby aubergines, but you can always use large ones and cut them into chunks if you prefer. This wonderful dish is so versatile that it even tastes great cold with a side salad.

SERVES 4 Ⓥ ❋
Syns per serving
Green: Free
Original: Free

EASY
Preparation time 5 minutes
Cooking time 30 minutes

Fry Light

2 tsp peeled and finely grated ginger

4 garlic cloves, peeled and crushed

1 tsp yellow mustard seeds

1 tsp cumin seeds

1 tsp black onion (nigella) seeds

1 tsp ground coriander

1 tsp ground cinnamon

1 tsp mild or medium curry powder

600g/1lb 6oz baby aubergines, halved lengthways

400g can chopped tomatoes

½ tsp artificial sweetener

salt

TO SERVE
large handful of freshly chopped coriander leaves

1. Spray a large non-stick frying pan with Fry Light and place over a high heat. Add the ginger, garlic, mustard seeds, cumin seeds and nigella and stir-fry for 2–3 minutes.

2. Then add the coriander, cinnamon, curry powder and aubergines and stir-fry for 1–2 minutes.

3. Add the tomatoes, sweetener and 100ml/3½fl oz of water and stir to mix well. Season with salt and bring to the boil. Then reduce the heat to low, cover and cook gently for 20–25 minutes, stirring often until the aubergines are tender. Remove from the heat and serve garnished with the chopped coriander.

COURGETTE CURRY

Fresh courgettes are cooked with tomatoes in this delicious curry, which makes a great lunch or dinner when served with rice and salads.

SERVES 4 Ⓥ ❄
Syns per serving
Green: Free
Original: Free

EASY
Preparation time 5 minutes
Cooking time 20 minutes

Fry Light
1 tsp cumin seeds
1 tsp black mustard seeds
1 onion, peeled, halved and thinly sliced
2 garlic cloves, peeled and crushed
1 tbsp mild or medium curry powder
700g/1lb 8oz courgettes, cut into slices or bite-sized cubes
400g can chopped tomatoes
1 tbsp tomato purée
½ tsp artificial sweetener
salt

TO SERVE
freshly chopped mint leaves
freshly chopped coriander leaves

1. Spray a large non-stick frying pan with Fry Light and place over a medium heat. Add the cumin and mustard seeds and when the seeds start to 'pop' add the onion and stir-fry for 5–6 minutes or until softened. Add the garlic, curry powder and courgette and cook for 3–4 minutes, stirring continuously.

2. Stir in the tomatoes, tomato purée, sweetener and 150ml/5fl oz of water and bring to the boil. Reduce the heat to low and cover, then simmer gently for 10–12 minutes.

3. Remove from the heat, season with salt, sprinkle over the chopped herbs and serve.

SPICED BEETROOT
WITH COCONUT

MEDIUM

This wonderful root vegetable is brought to life in this lightly spiced curry, which is made extra special with the addition of coconut milk.

SERVES 4 Ⓥ ❄

Syns per serving
Green: 2½
Original: 2½

EXTRA EASY
Preparation time 5 minutes
Cooking time 10 minutes

Fry Light

2 garlic cloves, peeled and crushed

1 tsp peeled and finely grated ginger

2 tsp cumin seeds

1 tsp coriander seeds, roughly crushed

1 dried red chilli, roughly crushed

700g/1lb 8oz beetroot, freshly cooked, peeled and cut into thick slices

150ml/5fl oz reduced-fat coconut milk

juice of 1 lime

zest of 1 lime, finely grated

½ tsp ground cardamom seeds

a small handful of coriander leaves, chopped

salt

1. Spray a large non-stick frying pan or wok with Fry Light and place over a high heat.

2. Add the garlic, ginger, cumin, coriander seeds and chilli and stir fry for 1–2 minutes.

3. Add the beetroot and stir-fry for 1–2 minutes. Then add the coconut milk, the juice and zest of the lime and the ground cardamom seeds. Cook for 2–3 minutes and then remove from the heat. Stir in the coriander leaves, season with salt and serve immediately.

TIP To cook fresh beetroot, either boil whole for 25–30 minutes until tender, then remove the skin, or bake them in a hot oven at 220°C/ Gas 7 for 25–30 minutes.
.

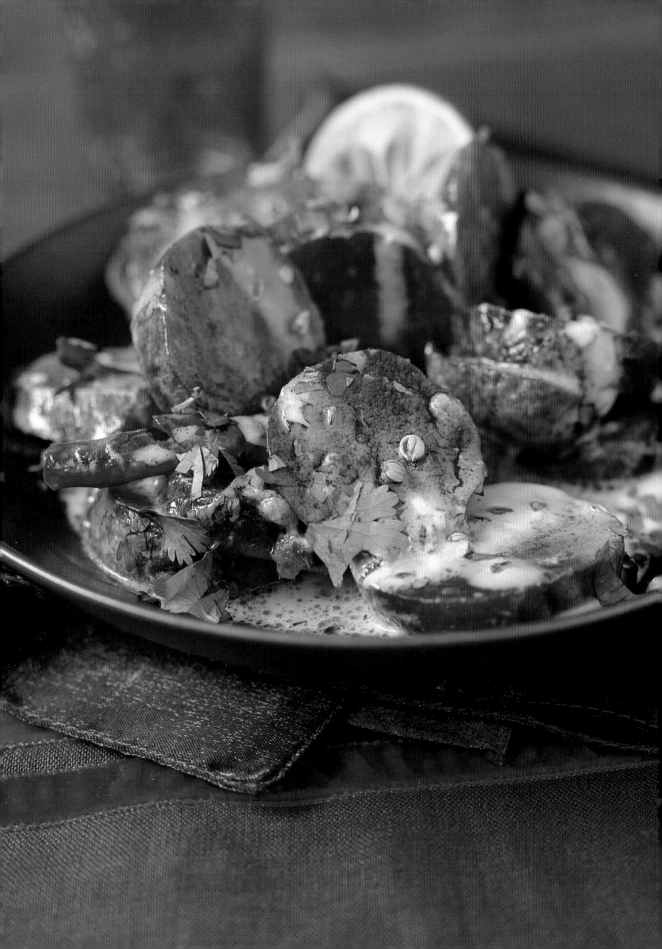

CURRIED
BUTTERNUT SQUASH

MEDIUM

In India, pumpkin is generally used for this recipe but butternut squash works just as well. This colourful dish is easy to cook and will become a regular on your Indian menu!

SERVES 4 Ⓥ ❄
Syns per serving
Green: Free
Original: Free

EASY
Preparation time 10 minutes
Cooking time 15 minutes

Fry Light

1 tsp fenugreek seeds

1 tsp turmeric

1 tsp dried red chilli, crushed

2 tsp coriander seeds, lightly crushed

1 butternut squash, peeled, deseeded and cut into bite-sized cubes

2 tsp fennel seeds, lightly crushed

1 tsp black peppercorns, crushed

1 tsp amchoor (dried mango powder) or 1 tbsp lemon juice if preferred

salt

1. Spray a large non-stick frying pan with Fry Light and place over a high heat. Add the fenugreek seeds to the pan and stir-fry for 15–20 seconds.

2. Then add the turmeric, chilli, coriander seeds and the squash and stir-fry for a further 3–4 minutes.

3. Pour about 250ml/9fl oz of boiling water into the pan and bring all the ingredients to the boil. Reduce the heat, cover and cook gently for 10–12 minutes. Then uncover and stir in the fennel, peppercorns and amchoor (or lemon juice) and continue to cook until most of the liquid has been absorbed and the squash is tender. Season well and serve.

GARAM MASALA TAMATAR

MEDIUM 🌶🌶

This dish is an old family favourite, using spiced tomatoes. It's a wonderful accompaniment to rice or eggs, and is best made with sweet and juicy tomatoes.

SERVES 4 Ⓥ ❄

Syns per serving
Green: Free
Original: Free

EASY
Preparation time 5 minutes
Cooking time 5 minutes

500g/1lb 2oz ripe tomatoes, halved
salt and freshly ground black pepper
½ tsp garam masala
2 tsp ground cumin
1 tsp cumin seeds
1 tsp mild chilli powder
2 tsp ground coriander
juice of 1–2 lemons

TO SERVE
freshly chopped mint leaves

1. Lay the tomato halves on a grill rack, cut side up.

2. Season well with the salt and black pepper. Mix together the garam masala, ground cumin, cumin seeds, chilli powder and coriander. Sprinkle this mixture evenly over the tomato halves.

3. Squeeze over the lemon juice and place the prepared grill rack under a hot grill, about 10cm/4in away from the grill source and grill for 5–6 minutes, or until the tops are lightly browned. Remove from the grill and garnish with the chopped mint leaves. Serve immediately.

ADRAKH SAAG BHAJI

MEDIUM 🌶🌶

Adrakh means 'ginger', and this wonderful dish of ginger and spinach is really easy to prepare and is packed full of goodness. To make it extra special, try using baby spinach leaves and make sure that the wok or frying pan is large enough to cope with the volume of spinach!

SERVES 4 Ⓥ
Syns per serving
Green: Free
Original: Free

EXTRA EASY
Preparation time 5 minutes
Cooking time 15 minutes

Fry Light

1 tbsp peeled and very finely shredded ginger

500g/1lb 2oz fresh spinach leaves, cleaned and trimmed

2 fresh green chillies, deseeded and finely chopped

½ tsp garam masala

½ tsp artificial sweetener

salt

1. Spray a large non-stick wok or frying pan with Fry Light and place over a medium heat. When hot enough, add the ginger and stir for 1–2 minutes until the ginger starts to go light brown.

2. Add the spinach and chilli and stir-fry for 6–7 minutes, stirring continuously, or until the spinach has wilted completely.

3. Then add the garam masala and sweetener and season well. Stir and cook for 2–3 minutes and remove from the heat. Serve immediately.

BANDH GOBI BHUNA

MILD ✎

This cabbage dish is full of flavour, and is simple yet effective. It's delicious served with any curry or is just as tasty on its own with some freshly boiled rice.

SERVES 4 Ⓥ ❄
Syns per serving
Green: Free
Original: Free

EASY
Preparation time 5 minutes
Cooking time 15 minutes

Fry Light

2 tsp cumin seeds

2 tsp fennel seeds

1 onion, peeled, halved and very thinly sliced

700g/1lb 8oz green cabbage, halved, cored and finely shredded

½ tsp mild chilli powder

½ tsp garam masala

salt

1. Spray a large non-stick frying pan with Fry Light and place over a high heat. Add the cumin and fennel seeds to the pan and stir-fry for 30–40 seconds.

2. Add the onion and stir-fry for 5–6 minutes or until the onion starts to go light brown.

3. Then add the cabbage and continue to stir-fry over a high heat or until the cabbage starts to wilt and lightly brown. Add the chilli powder and turn the heat to low. Cook for 7–8 minutes, stirring often. Sprinkle in the garam masala and season well. Remove from the heat and serve.

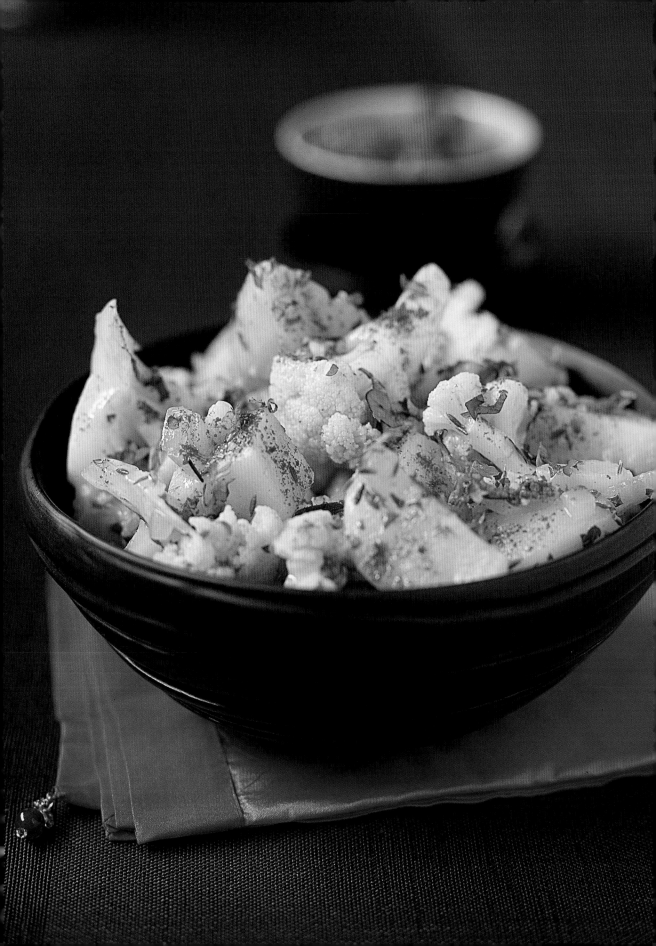

ALOO GOBI

MEDIUM ♪♪

A favourite restaurant speciality, this potato and cauliflower dish is gently spiced and makes a great supper when served on a bed of rice with a side salad.

SERVES 4 Ⓥ ❋
Syns per serving
Green: Free
EASY
Preparation time 5 minutes
Cooking time 30 minutes

Fry Light

1 onion, peeled and finely chopped

2 tsp cumin seeds

2 large potatoes, peeled and cut into bite-sized cubes

1 head of cauliflower, cut into bite-sized florets

1 tsp mild or medium chilli powder

½ tsp turmeric

2 tsp ground coriander

2 tsp garam masala

2 tsp amchoor (dried mango powder)

salt

TO SERVE
freshly chopped coriander leaves
freshly chopped mint leaves

1. Spray a large non-stick wok with Fry Light and place over a medium heat. Add the onion to the wok and stir-fry for 4–5 minutes until softened. Add the cumin seeds and stir-fry for a further 2–3 minutes.

2. Add the potatoes and cauliflower and stir-fry over a high heat for 4–5 minutes. Add the chilli powder, turmeric, ground coriander, garam masala and amchoor and stir-fry for 2–3 minutes.

3. Pour in 200ml/7fl oz of water and season well. Cover and cook gently for 10–15 minutes, or until the cauliflower and potatoes are tender. Season to taste. Remove from the heat and serve garnished with the chopped herbs.

SUKKI GOBI

MEDIUM 🌶🌶

Sukki means 'dry' and here the cauliflower florets are cooked to perfection in this aromatic stir-fry. If you prefer, you can use broccoli as an alternative to the cauliflower.

SERVES 4 (V) ❄

Syns per serving
Green: Free
Original: Free

EXTRA EASY
Preparation time 5 minutes
Cooking time 10 minutes

Fry Light

1 tsp cumin seeds

1 tsp yellow mustard seeds

3 garlic cloves, peeled and finely chopped

1 tbsp peeled and finely shredded ginger

500g/1lb 2oz cauliflower florets

1 fresh green chilli, deseeded and finely chopped

salt and freshly ground black pepper

½ tsp garam masala

TO SERVE
lemon wedges

1. Spray a large non-stick wok with Fry Light and place over a high heat. Add the cumin and mustard seeds.

2. As soon as the seeds start to 'pop', add the garlic, ginger, cauliflower and chilli. Stir-fry for 6–7 minutes until the florets are lightly browned.

3. Season with salt and pepper, add the garam masala and 4–5 tablespoons of water, toss to mix well, then cover and cook for 2–3 minutes. Serve immediately with the lemon wedges squeezed over.

PHOOL GOBI

MEDIUM ✔✔

Another popular dry curry, this tastes great served with rice or lentils. This dish can also be prepared quickly, which is great after a long day at work!

SERVES 4 Ⓥ ❋
Syns per serving
Green: Free
Original: 1

EASY
Preparation time 5 minutes
Cooking time 25 minutes

Fry Light

2 tsp cumin seeds

1 small onion, peeled and finely chopped

1 fresh green chilli, deseeded and finely sliced

2 plum tomatoes, roughly chopped

1 tsp mild or medium chilli powder

1 tsp garam masala

1 tsp ground cumin

1 tsp ground coriander

½ tsp turmeric

½ tsp artificial sweetener

1 tbsp lemon juice

400g/14oz carrots, peeled and cut into 2cm/¾in cubes

400g/14oz cauliflower, broken into small florets

110g/4oz fresh or frozen peas

2 tbsp very low fat natural yogurt

salt

1. Spray a large non-stick frying pan with Fry Light and place over a medium heat. Add the cumin seeds and onion and stir-fry for 4–5 minutes or until the onion is soft.

2. Add the chilli, tomatoes, chilli powder, garam masala, cumin and coriander, turmeric, sweetener and lemon juice and then add 100ml/3½fl oz of water and cook gently for 3–4 minutes.

3. Add the carrots, cauliflower and peas. Stir, cover and simmer gently for 10–12 minutes, stirring occasionally, until tender. Remove from the heat, stir in the yogurt, season well and serve immediately.

TIP If you don't have all the spices, swap them for 1–2 tbsp mild curry powder.

MAKKAI-LAL MIRCH BHAJI

MEDIUM 🌶🌶

Tender yellow sweetcorn kernels are cooked with red peppers and tomatoes in this tasty vegetarian curry. You can use canned sweetcorn kernels if you want to, but it is always better to use fresh corn, if it's available.

SERVES 4 Ⓥ ❋
Syns per serving
Green: Free

EASY
Preparation time 5 minutes
Cooking time 20 minutes

2 fresh corn-on-the-cob
Fry Light
1 small onion, finely chopped
2 red peppers, deseeded and cut into 2cm/¾in cubes
1 fresh green chilli, cut in half lengthways and deseeded
6–8 fresh curry leaves
1 tsp ground coriander
250g/9oz chopped tomatoes
½ tsp artificial sweetener
3 tbsp finely chopped coriander leaves
1 tsp garam masala
salt

TO SERVE
lemon wedges

1. Using a sharp knife, strip the corn kernels off the cobs, put into a bowl and set aside.

2. Spray a large non-stick frying pan with Fry Light and place over a medium heat. Add the onion and stir-fry for 4–5 minutes until softened.

3. Add the sweetcorn, red pepper, chilli, curry leaves and ground coriander and stir-fry for 2 minutes. Then add the tomatoes and sweetener, stir, cover and cook gently for 8–10 minutes.

4. Remove the frying pan from the heat and stir in the chopped coriander and garam masala. Season well and serve with the lemon wedges squeezed over.

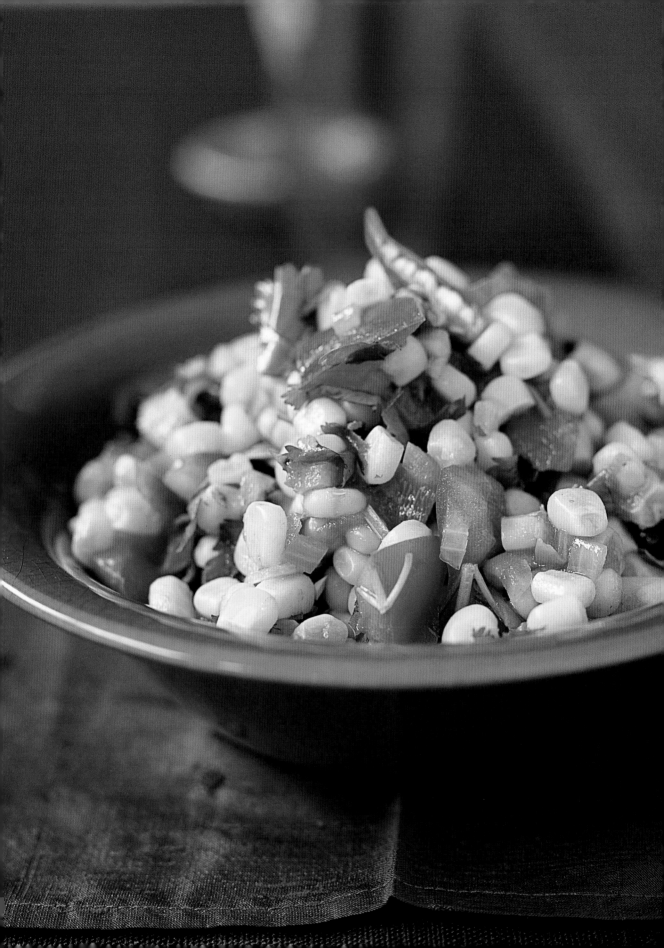

EEDAA PER BROCCOLI

This is a simple dish that is usually cooked with potatoes but here we've decided to use broccoli florets as an alternative. This dish is also quick and easy so is perfect for a midweek family supper.

SERVES 4 Ⓥ ❄
Syns per serving
Green: Free
Original: Free
EASY
Preparation time 5 minutes
Cooking time 10 minutes

Fry Light

1 red onion, peeled, halved and very thinly sliced

1 fresh green chilli, deseeded and finely chopped

½ tsp turmeric

2 tsp ground cumin

1 tsp ground coriander

450g/1lb broccoli, cut into small florets

salt and freshly ground black pepper

4 large eggs, lightly beaten

2 tbsp finely chopped coriander

2 tbsp deseeded and finely diced red pepper

1. Spray a large non-stick frying pan with Fry Light and place over a medium heat. Add the onion and chilli to the pan and stir-fry for 3–4 minutes.

2. Add the turmeric, ground cumin and coriander and stir-fry for 20–30 seconds. Then add the broccoli and season well. Increase the heat to high and stir-fry for 2–3 minutes.

3. Mix the eggs with the chopped coriander and diced pepper. Season well and pour the eggs over the broccoli mixture. Stir for 2–3 minutes or until you have a soft scrambled egg mixture coating the broccoli. Remove from the heat and serve.

SPICED ROASTED SWEDE

Swedes, tubers and other root vegetables are eaten widely across the length and breadth of India. In this recipe, pieces of swede are tossed with spices and roasted in the oven until deliciously tender. Why not try substituting celeriac for the swede for another tasty option?

SERVES 4 Ⓥ ❄

Syns per serving
Green: Free
Original: Free

EXTRA EASY
Preparation time 5 minutes
Cooking time 25 minutes

Fry Light
1 tsp ground cumin
1 tsp ground coriander
1 tsp ground cinnamon
2 tsp cumin seeds
2 tsp coriander seeds, crushed
2 tsp dried red chilli, crushed
2 tsp black mustard seeds
700g/1lb 8oz swede, peeled and cut into thick batons
juice of 2 lemons
salt

1. Preheat the oven to 220°C/Gas 7. Line a baking sheet with non-stick baking parchment and spray with Fry Light.

2. Mix together the spices and dust over the swede pieces. Add the lemon juice and toss to coat evenly. Arrange the swede pieces in a single layer on the prepared baking sheet, season with salt and spray with Fry Light.

3. Place in the oven and roast for 15–20 minutes or until tender and lightly charred at the edges. Remove from the oven and serve.

TIP Swap the ground cumin, coriander and cinnamon and the cumin and coriander seeds for 2 tablespoons of mild or medium curry powder if desired.

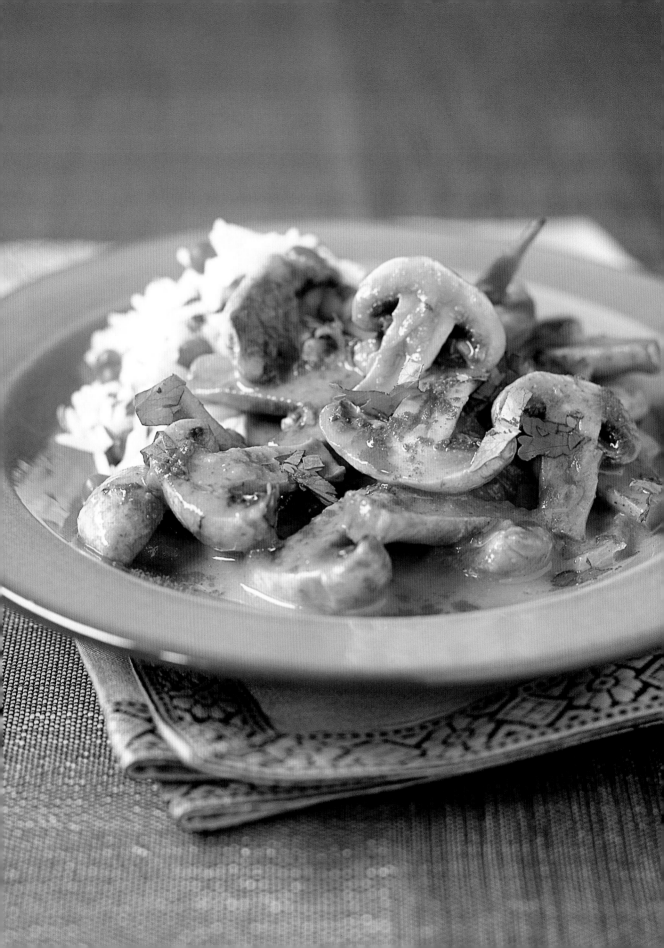

KHUMBI CURRY

This is a quick and easy curry that uses button mushrooms as the main ingredient. If you prefer, you can use any seasonal mushrooms or dried mushrooms that have been re-hydrated.

SERVES 4 Ⓥ ❄

Syns per serving
Green: Free
Original: Free

EASY
Preparation time 5 minutes
Cooking time 15 minutes

2 tsp peeled and finely grated ginger

110g/4oz onion, peeled and finely grated

4 garlic cloves, peeled and crushed

Fry Light

500g/1lb 2oz large button mushrooms, halved or quartered

3 tbsp very low fat natural yogurt

1 tbsp tomato purée

2 tsp ground coriander

1 tsp mild chilli powder

salt and freshly ground black pepper

4 tbsp chopped coriander leaves

1. Mix together the ginger, onion and garlic with 4 tablespoons of water in a small bowl and set aside.

2. Spray a large non-stick wok with Fry Light and place over a high heat. Add the mushrooms and stir-fry for 5–6 minutes or until lightly browned. Transfer the mushrooms to a bowl and set aside. Wipe the wok with sheets of kitchen paper and re-spray with Fry Light.

3. Place over a high heat and add the onion mixture. Stir-fry for 3–4 minutes and then add the yogurt, 1 tablespoon at a time. Add the tomato purée and ground coriander and stir-fry for 1 minute before adding 300ml/½ pint of water, the mushrooms with juices and the chilli powder.

4. Season well and simmer gently for 5–6 minutes (do not boil). Remove from the heat and stir in the chopped coriander. If you're following the Green choice serve with Pea pilau (see page 165).

MUMBAI ALOO

A terrific partnership of flavours and textures, these cumin-scented potatoes are a perfect match for the taste buds. If you're in a rush, you could always use cooked, leftover potatoes.

SERVES 4 Ⓥ ❄

Syns per serving
Green: Free

EASY

Preparation time 5 minutes
Cooking time 25 minutes

900g/2lb potatoes (Desiree or King Edwards), peeled and cut into cubes

salt

Fry Light

2 tsp cumin seeds

1 tsp ground cumin

1 tsp ground coriander

½ tsp garam masala

½ tsp mild or medium chilli powder

4–5 tbsp finely chopped coriander leaves

1. Boil the potato cubes in a pan of lightly salted water for 10 minutes or until just tender. Drain thoroughly and set aside.

2. Spray a large non-stick wok or frying pan with Fry Light and place over a medium-high heat. Add the cumin seeds and stir-fry for 1–2 minutes. Add the potatoes and cook until lightly browned on all sides.

3. Turn the heat to low. Then add the ground cumin, ground coriander, garam masala and chilli powder. Season well and cook for a further 1–2 minutes. Remove from the heat and stir in the chopped coriander. Serve immediately.

TIP This dish would work equally well with parsnips, butternut squash, swede or celeriac.

INDIAN-STYLE SPICY
MASHED POTATOES

MEDIUM ✔✔

Here's a twist on the classic mashed potato. It's made with fresh herbs and spices and creates a wonderful dish that is a great accompaniment to any curry or is terrific on its own served with a side salad.

SERVES 4 Ⓥ ❅

Syns per serving
Green: Free

EXTRA EASY
Preparation time 5 minutes
Cooking time 15 minutes

1kg/2lb 4oz potatoes (Desiree or King Edwards), peeled and cut into cubes

salt

200g pot very low fat natural yogurt

4 spring onions, trimmed and very finely sliced

1 fresh red chilli, deseeded and finely sliced

a large handful of chopped coriander leaves

2 plum tomatoes, deseeded and finely diced

1 tbsp lemon juice

½ tsp ground cumin

½ tsp ground coriander

½ tsp mild or medium chilli powder

1. Place the potatoes in a large saucepan of lightly salted water. Bring to the boil and cook for 12–15 minutes or until the potatoes are tender.

2. Drain the potatoes and return to the pan. Then mash using a potato masher.

3. Stir in the yogurt and mix well. Add the remaining ingredients, season well with salt and serve.

SAAG DAHI KARI

This is a wonderful curry from Kashmir in northern India, where the vegetables are cooked in a spicy, aromatic yogurt sauce.

SERVES 4 Ⓥ ❄

Syns per serving
Green: 1
Original: 1½

EASY

Preparation time 5 minutes
Cooking time 20 minutes

Fry Light

2 fresh green chillies, deseeded and finely chopped

1 tsp peeled and finely grated ginger

2 tsp ground cumin

1 tsp black peppercorns, crushed

1 tsp ground cinnamon

1 tsp ground cardamom seeds

a pinch of grated nutmeg

400g packet Free mixed vegetables (see Free Food list on page 218)

25g/1oz peas

150g pot very low fat natural yogurt

150ml/5fl oz vegetable stock made with Vecon

salt

TO SERVE

1 tbsp flaked almonds

1. Spray a large non-stick frying pan with Fry Light and place over a medium heat. Add the chilli and ginger and stir-fry for 2–3 minutes. Add the remaining spices and stir-fry for a further 2–3 minutes.

2. Add the mixed vegetables and peas and stir-fry for 3–4 minutes.

3. Blend the yogurt with the stock and add to the pan. Stir, cover and cook gently for 10–12 minutes (do not allow to boil) or until the vegetables are just tender. Season and garnish with the flaked almonds.

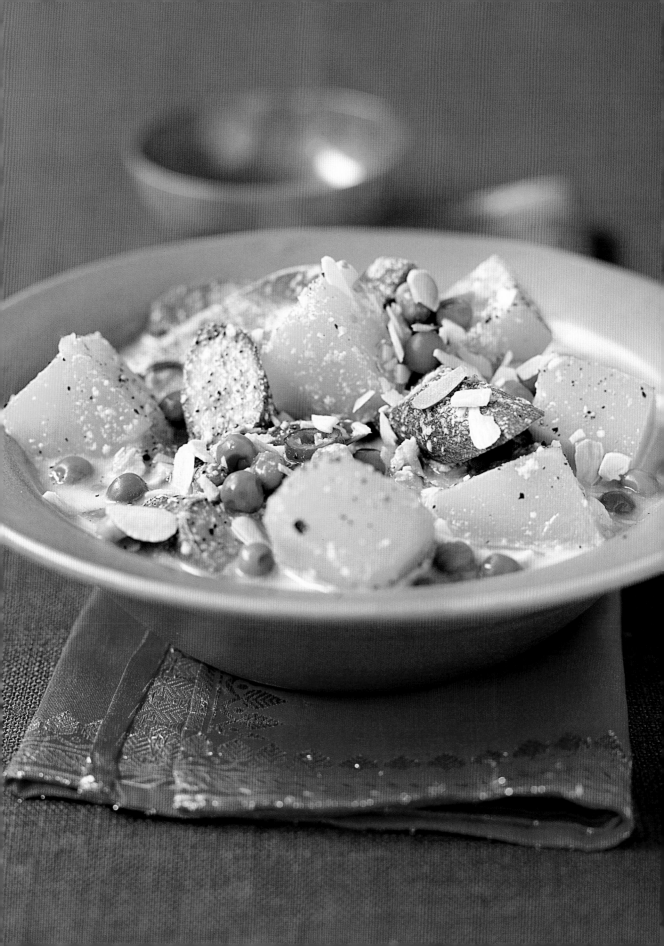

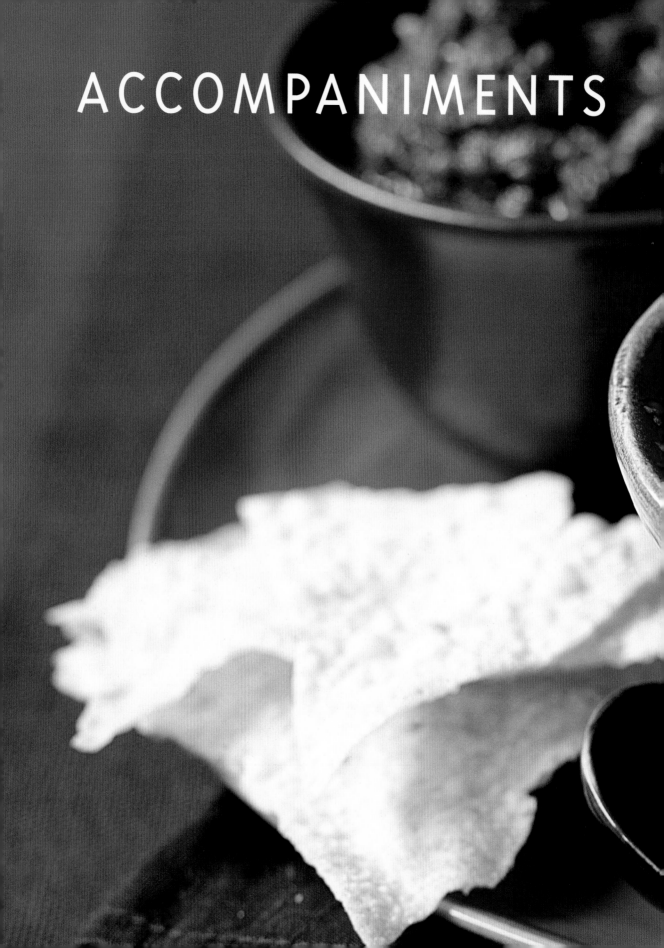

ACCOMPANIMENTS

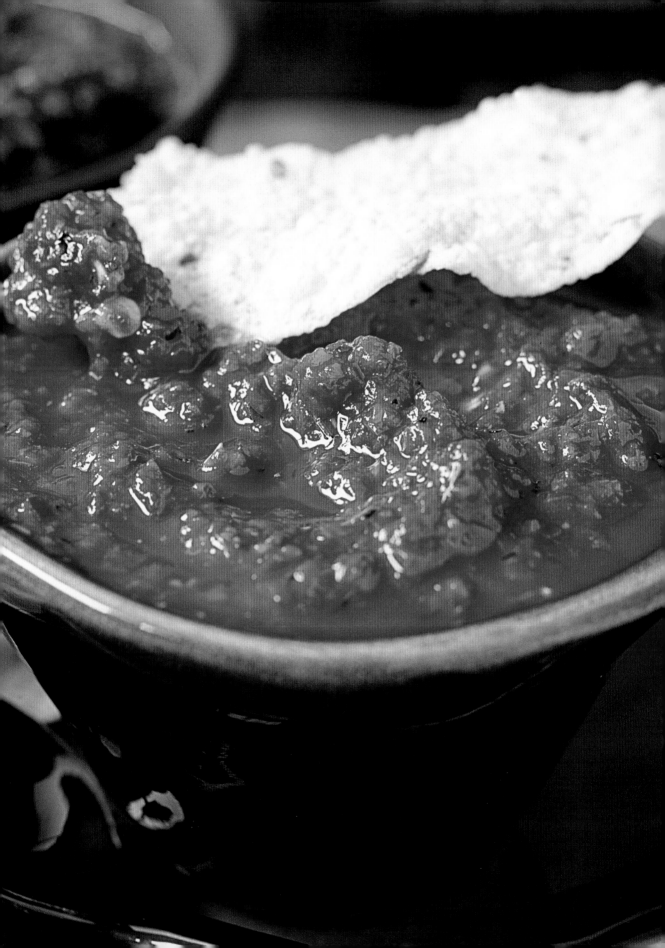

BRINJAL BHARTA

This smoky-flavoured aubergine dip is a favourite from the state of Punjab. It is wonderful also when used as a spread or filling for sandwiches and will keep in an airtight jar in the fridge for up to a week.

SERVES 4 Ⓥ ❋
Syns per serving
Green: Free
Original: Free

WORTH THE EFFORT
Preparation time 5 minutes
Cooking time 30 minutes
(plus chilling)

2 large aubergines

1 tsp peeled and finely grated ginger

1 garlic clove, peeled and crushed

1 fresh green chilli, deseeded and finely sliced

1 tsp ground cumin

1 tsp ground coriander

2 tsp tomato purée

4–5 tbsp very low fat natural yogurt

a small handful of chopped coriander leaves

salt

1. Preheat the oven to 220°C/Gas 7. Prick the aubergines all over with a skewer and place on a baking tray. Cook in the oven for 30 minutes or until collapsed. Remove and allow to cool completely.

2. Halve the aubergine lengthways and carefully scoop out all of the flesh and place in a food processor together with all the accumulated juices.

3. Add the ginger, garlic, chilli, cumin, ground coriander, tomato purée and yogurt and blend until fairly smooth. Transfer to a mixing bowl, stir in the chopped coriander, season well and chill for 3–4 hours to allow the flavours to develop before serving.

MOOLI-GAJJAR RAITA

MILD ⟋

A twist on the classic coleslaw, this colourful relish uses mooli (white radish) and carrots mixed together with cooling yogurt and fresh herbs to give you a perfect foil to any fiery or spicy dish. Mooli is now widely available in supermarkets but if unavailable, use thinly sliced red radish or cabbage instead.

SERVES 4 Ⓥ
Syns per serving
Green: Free
Original: Free

EASY
Preparation time 10 minutes
(plus chilling)
Cooking time none

150g pot very low fat natural yogurt

2 tbsp finely chopped mint leaves

2 tbsp finely chopped coriander leaves

½ small red onion, peeled and thinly sliced

¼ tsp ground cumin

salt and freshly ground black pepper

1 mooli (white radish), peeled and coarsely grated

2 carrots, peeled and coarsely grated

1. In a mixing bowl, whisk the yogurt until smooth and then stir in the chopped herbs, red onion, cumin and seasoning.

2. Fold in the grated radish and carrot and stir to mix well. Cover and chill in the fridge for 20–30 minutes before serving.

LA SIMLA MIRCH CHUTNEY

MEDIUM 🌶🌶

This extremely easy red pepper chutney can be prepared in a flash and goes well with almost any dish. Once made, it will keep in the fridge for 3–4 days. You can also freeze it for up to a month.

SERVES 4 Ⓥ ❄

Syns per serving
Green: Free
Original: Free

EXTRA EASY
Preparation time 10 minutes
(plus chilling)
Cooking time none

1 red pepper, roasted, skinned, deseeded and finely chopped

6 tbsp chopped mint leaves

juice of 1 lemon

1 garlic clove, peeled and finely sliced

1 fresh red chilli, deseeded and finely sliced

2 tbsp finely chopped dill

salt

1. Place the red pepper, mint, lemon juice and garlic in a food processor.

2. Add the chilli, dill and a little salt and blend until fairly smooth, but still a little chunky.

3. Transfer to a bowl and chill until ready to use.

NOTE The dish at the front of the photograph is La simla mirch chutney; that at the back is Hara chutney (see recipe on page 210).

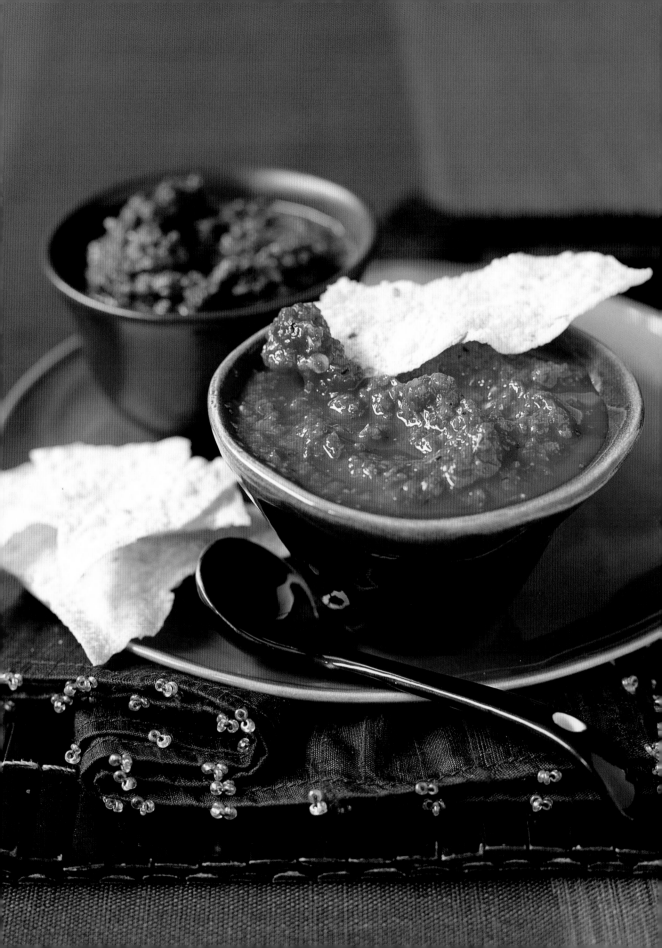

HARA CHUTNEY

HOT 🌶🌶🌶

This fragrant chutney, made from fresh coriander, mint, ginger, garlic and spices, is the perfect accompaniment to any Indian meal and is also wonderful spread on grilled fish or meat. It will keep in the fridge for a week if well sealed.

SERVES 4 Ⓥ ❄

Syns per serving
Green: Free
Original: Free

EXTRA EASY
Preparation time 5 minutes
Cooking time none

110g/4oz coriander leaves, finely chopped

50g/2oz mint leaves, finely chopped

1 tsp peeled and finely grated ginger

2 fresh green chillies, finely chopped

juice of 2 limes

2 tsp sea salt

¼ tsp artificial sweetener

1. Place all the ingredients in a food processor with 75ml/2½fl oz of water and blend until smooth.

2. You can use this chutney immediately or you can store it in an airtight jar or container in the fridge for up to seven days.

CUCUMBER, CHILLI AND MINT RAITA

MILD ✦

Cool, fresh and tasty, this raita makes an ideal accompaniment to any dish, snack or meal.

SERVES 4 ⓥ
Syns per serving
Green: Free
Original: Free

EASY
Preparation time 10 minutes
Cooking time none

1 large cucumber, peeled, deseeded and coarsely grated

250g/9oz very low fat natural yogurt

¼ tsp artificial sweetener

1 fresh red chilli, deseeded and finely chopped

8 tbsp finely chopped mint leaves

juice of ½ lime

2 tsp roasted cumin seeds

1–2 tsp sea salt

1. Place the cucumber in a fine sieve and squeeze out all the liquid from it and place it in a bowl.

2. Add the yogurt, sweetener, chilli, mint, lime juice and cumin seeds to the bowl and stir to mix well.

3. Season well and chill for 20–30 minutes before serving.

KACHUMBER

This diced tomato, cucumber and onion salad is the ultimate accompaniment to any Indian meal. Simple and really easy to put together, it benefits from standing at room temperature for 10–15 minutes before serving to allow the flavours to develop.

SERVES 4 Ⓥ
Syns per serving
Green: Free
Original: Free

EASY
Preparation time 10 minutes
(plus chilling)
Cooking time none

1 cucumber, peeled, deseeded
and finely diced

4 firm plum tomatoes, deseeded
and finely diced

½ onion, peeled and finely diced

4 tbsp chopped coriander leaves

2 tbsp chopped mint leaves

juice of 2 limes

salt and freshly ground black
pepper

1. Place the cucumber, tomatoes and onion in a mixing bowl and add the chopped herbs.

2. Add the juice of the limes and season well. Stir to mix and allow to sit at room temperature for 10–15 minutes to allow the flavours to develop before serving.

KHATTA-MEETTA
TAMATAR CHUTNEY

This spiced sweet tomato relish makes a great accompaniment to any Indian meal. Once made, it will keep in the fridge for up to a week.

SERVES 4 Ⓥ ❄
Syns per serving
Green: Free
Original: Free

EASY
Preparation time 5 minutes
Cooking time 30 minutes
(plus chilling)

Fry Light

1 onion, peeled, halved and thinly sliced

1 tsp peeled and finely grated ginger

1 tsp crushed dried red chillies

2 tsp black mustard seeds

2 tsp cumin seeds

1 tsp crushed coriander seeds

3 garlic cloves, peeled and thinly sliced

6 plum tomatoes, skinned and roughly chopped

2 tsp artificial sweetener

salt

6 tbsp finely chopped coriander leaves

1. Spray a frying pan with Fry Light and place over a medium heat. Add the onion to the pan and gently fry for 6–7 minutes or until lightly browned.

2. Add the ginger, dried chilli, mustard, cumin and coriander seeds and the garlic. Stir and cook for 2–3 minutes.

3. Stir in the tomatoes and sweetener and cook gently for 15–20 minutes, stirring constantly. Season well and then remove from the heat. Stir in the chopped coriander and allow to cool before serving. If you are going to store the chutney, place it in a sterilised jar, seal well and chill in the fridge for up to a week.

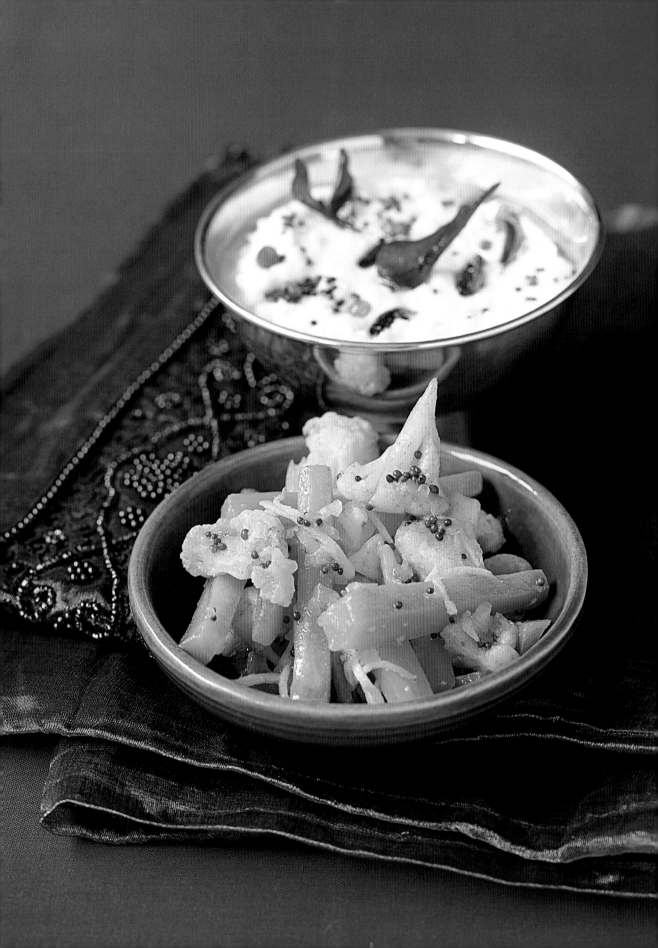

GAJJAR PHOOL GOBI AACHAR

MEDIUM

This tart, spicy and sweet pickle is made using carrots and cauliflower. It needs about 8–10 days to mature before you use it.

SERVES 4 (V)
Syns per serving
Green: Free
Original: Free

WORTH THE EFFORT
Preparation time 10 minutes
Cooking time 4 hours
(plus drying and maturing)

3 carrots, scrubbed and chopped into small bite-sized pieces

110g/4oz small cauliflower florets

4 tbsp white wine vinegar

1 tsp artificial sweetener

Fry Light

2 tbsp peeled and finely grated onion

1 tbsp peeled and finely grated ginger

1 tsp peeled and finely grated garlic

2 tbsp roughly ground black mustard seeds

4 tsp sea salt

2 tsp mild or medium coarse red chilli powder

1 tsp turmeric

1 tsp garam masala

1. Place the vegetables in a steamer and steam for 3–4 minutes. Remove and drain thoroughly on kitchen paper. Spread the vegetables on a baking tray lined with baking parchment. Preheat your oven to the lowest setting and place the baking tray in the oven for 3–4 hours to dry out. Remove from the oven and place the vegetables on a clean, dry baking sheet and leave to dry out completely overnight.

2. Place the vinegar in a small bowl and add the sweetener. Stir to dissolve and set aside.

3. Spray a frying pan with Fry Light and place over a medium heat. Add the onion, ginger and garlic and stir and cook gently until lightly browned. Add the remaining spices and prepared vegetables, stir and remove from the heat. Pour over the vinegar mixture and stir to mix well.

4. Pack the pickle into a small, sterilised jar, seal tightly and shake vigorously to combine. Leave to mature for 8–10 days, shaking the jar every other day to mix.

NOTE The dish at the front of the photograph is Gajjar phool gobi aachar; that at the back is Naryal chutney (see recipe on page 216).

NARYAL CHUTNEY

This is a typical southern Indian relish made from freshly grated coconut. You can, however, substitute dried, desiccated coconut in this recipe (soak it in warm water for 20 minutes and drain before use). Yogurt and spices make this a lovely zesty accompaniment to any Indian meal. It has to be used on the day it is made.

SERVES 4 ⓥ
Syns per serving
Green: 1½
Original: 1½

EASY
Preparation time 10 minutes
Cooking time 5 minutes

25g/1oz fresh coconut, finely grated

6 tbsp very low fat natural yogurt, lightly beaten

Fry Light

2 tsp black mustard seeds

10 fresh curry leaves

1 fresh green chilli, deseeded and sliced

1 tsp peeled and finely grated ginger

2 tsp split Bengal gram (channa dal) (optional)

2 small dried red chillies

1 tsp sea salt

1. Mix the coconut and yogurt together to create a rough paste.

2. Spray a frying pan with Fry Light and place over a medium heat. Add the mustard seeds and when they start to 'pop', add the curry leaves, green chilli, ginger, gram (if using) and dried red chilli. Stir-fry for 1 minute.

3. Scrape the contents of the frying pan into the coconut mixture, add the salt and stir to mix well.

TIP If you can't find Bengal gram, you can substitute it for yellow split peas.

LIME PICKLE

This classic pickle is a doddle to make and is a wonderful way to enliven any meal. Try to find thin-skinned limes for this pickle, to facilitate the spices permeating the fruit more easily. Once made, this pickle can be stored for months if kept in a cool place.

SERVES 4 Ⓥ

Syns per serving
Green: Free
Original: Free

WORTH THE EFFORT
Preparation time 10 minutes
(plus soaking and standing)
Cooking time none

8 small thin-skinned limes

6 tsp sea salt

2 tsp mild or medium coarse red chilli powder

2 tsp cumin seeds

2 tsp freshly ground black pepper

2 tsp garam masala

2 tbsp artificial sweetener

1. Place seven of the limes in a bowl and cover with cold water. Leave to soak at room temperature for 3–4 days and drain.

2. Halve the limes, roughly chop into small bite-sized pieces and place in a bowl. Mix the remaining ingredients together, add to the bowl and, using your fingers, mix well to coat evenly.

3. Pack the pieces of lime tightly in a small, sterilised container and squeeze over the juice of the remaining lime. Seal the jar and shake well to combine. Leave to stand for a month, shaking the jar every other day.

FREE FOOD SELECTION

We have listed many of our Free Foods here. For the full list, you will need to become a Slimming World member.

* Foods marked with an **S** symbol **will give your weight loss a boost**. Choosing foods marked with an **SS** symbol will give your weight loss an even **bigger boost**.
* Foods marked with **F** will give you **extra fibre** and those marked **FF** will give you an even **richer helping of fibre**.
* Foods marked **H** will keep you **healthy** and those marked **HH** are **vital to your health** and need to be included in your diet **every day**.

S	= weight loss boost
SS	= extra weight loss boost
F	= extra fibre
FF	= extra-rich fibre
H	= healthy
HH	= vital to health

GREEN CHOICE FREE FOODS

All vegetables are classed as a Free Food when on a Green day.

The following fruits can be eaten freely as long as they are fresh or frozen varieties.

Grains, Pulses & Vegetables

Bulgar wheat			H
Couscous			H
Dried Pasta			H
Rice, all types			H
Baked beans	SS	F	H
Chickpeas		F	H
Lentils	S	F	H
Peas	SS	F	H
Red kidney beans	S	FF	H
Soya beans		FF	H
Potatoes			HH
Quorn	SS	F	H
Tofu			

Dairy

Eggs		
Very low fat natural cottage cheese		H
Very low fat natural fromage frais	H	
Very low fat natural yogurt		H

Fruit

Apples	S		HH
Apricots	S		HH
Bananas			HH
Blackberries	SS	F	HH
Blueberries			HH
Cherries	S		HH
Grapefruit	SS		HH
Grapes			HH
Kiwi fruit	S		HH
Mango			HH
Melon	SS		HH
Nectarines	S		HH
Oranges	S		HH
Papaya	S		HH
Peaches	S		HH
Pears	S		HH
Pineapple	S		HH
Plums	S		HH
Raspberries	SS		HH
Strawberries	SS		HH

ORIGINAL CHOICE FREE FOODS

Not all vegetables are Free Foods on the Original Choice. Choose freely from the following list:

Vegetables

Asparagus	S		HH
Aubergine	S		HH
Baby whole sweetcorn	S		HH
Beans, French/green	S	F	HH
Beetroot	S		HH
Broccoli	S	F	HH
Brussels sprouts	S	F	HH
Cabbage	S		HH
Carrots	S		HH
Cauliflower	S		HH
Courgettes	S		HH
Cucumber	S		HH
Mushrooms	S		HH
Onions	S		HH
Peppers	S		HH
Salad leaves	S		HH
Spinach	S		HH
Spring onions	S		HH
Squash	S		HH
Sugar snap peas	S		HH
Swede	S		HH
Tomatoes	S		HH
Quorn	SS	F	H
Tofu			

Poultry (skin removed)

Chicken	S	H
Turkey	S	H

Meat (all visible fat removed)

Bacon
Beef
Ham
Lamb
Pork

Fish

Cod	SS	H
Haddock	SS	H
Kippers		H
Mackerel (*not smoked*)		H
Pilchards		H
Plaice	SS	H
Salmon (*fresh, canned and smoked*)		H
Sole	SS	H

Shellfish

Crab		H
Prawns	S	H

Dairy

Eggs	
Very low fat natural cottage cheese	H
Very low fat natural fromage frais	H
Very low fat natural yogurt	H

The following fruits can be eaten freely as long as they are fresh or frozen varieties.

Fruit

Apples	S		HH
Apricots	S		HH
Bananas			HH
Blackberries	SS	F	HH
Blueberries			HH
Cherries	S		HH
Grapefruit	SS		HH
Grapes			HH
Kiwi fruit	S		HH
Mango			HH
Melon	SS		HH
Nectarines	S		HH
Oranges	S		HH
Papaya	S		HH
Peaches	S		HH
Pears	S		HH
Pineapple	S		HH
Plums	S		HH
Raspberries	SS		HH
Strawberries	SS		HH

SYNS SELECTION

Listed below is a selection of Syn values for foods that you can enjoy every day. The values apply to both the Green and Original choices.

Alcohol

25ml/1fl oz measure of any spirit	2½
150ml/5fl oz glass of wine	5
300ml/½ pint beer/lager	5
300ml/½ pint cider	5

Biscuits and Bars each

Cheese thin/water biscuit	1
Chocolate finger	1½
Jacob's Essentials Crackers, per triangle	1½
Fruit shortcake/rich tea	2
Cream cracker	2
Jaffa cake/ginger nut	2½
Custard cream	3
Quaker Snack-a-Jacks Jumbo Delight	3½
Chocolate digestive/jammie dodger	4
Kellogg's Special K Cereal Bar	4½
McVities Penguin Bar	7

Cakes each

Cadbury Mini Roll	5½
Mr Kipling French Fancy	5½
Mr Kipling Country/Lemon Slice	6
McVities Jaffa Cake Cake Bar	6½
Cadbury Irresistibles Cake Bar	7½
Mr Kipling Angel/Bakewell Slice	7½

Chocolates and Sweets standard bag/tube etc

Milky Bar	3½
Fun-size bars	5
2 finger Kit Kat	5½
Fudge/Milky Way	6
Curly Wurly	6½
Polo Mints	7
Fruit Gums	8
Flake/Maltesers	9
Fruit Pastilles	10

Crisps standard bag

French Fries/Golden Lights	4½
Potato Heads/Quavers	5
Ryvita Minis	5
Seasons Crispbread Snacks	6
Special K Lite Bites	6
Snack-a-jacks	7

Desserts per pot

Müllerlight Fruit Halo	4½
Rowntree's Ready to Eat Jelly Pot	5
Cadbury Light Chocolate Mousse (100g pot)	5½
Müllerice, Only 1% Fat	6
Danone Goodies Trifle	7
Onken Lite Mousse	8

Ice Creams/Lollies

Fruit Pastil Ice Lolly/Mini Calippo	3
50g/2oz scoop low fat ice cream	4
Fab Ice Lolly	4
Solero	5
Skinny Cow Ice Cream Cone	6
Magnum Light	8½

Nuts per 25g/1oz

Cashew nuts, shelled	8
Peanuts, salted	8½
Brazil nuts, shelled	9½
Walnuts, shelled	10

Sauces and Spreads

Aerosol cream: 2 level tbsp	½
Custard made with skimmed milk: 2 level tbsp	1
Gravy made without fat: 4 level tbsp	1
Reduced calorie mayonnaise: 1 level tbsp	2½
Margarine/spread, low fat variety: 25g/1oz	5½
Oil, any variety: 1 level tbsp	6

INDEX